My Health

Taking Control of Your Personal Healthcare

Fairhaven Media

FAIRHAVEN MEDIA

MY HEALTH
Copyright 2022 © by Hubert and Sheila Robertson

Cover by: Izzit Graphics *www.izzitgraphics.com*
Interior Layout: Sheila Robertson

Printed in the United States of America

ISBN: 978-1-947729-10-0
Personal Health, Health record, Dental

This book is all about you and your health. As a log book of doctor's visits, procedures, prescriptions and other valuable information, you will always have pertinent health facts at your fingertips.

Start filling in your information today and as you move forward on your journey of health you can add to your personal health profile.

This book is the health history of:

_____

This book of health history was started on:

_____
date

_____
age

INDEX

General Health Info

Name_____

Date of Birth _____

Birth weight:_____   Birth length: _____

Condition at birth (i.e. healthy, premature, medical issues):

_____

_____

_____

_____

_____

Childhood Conditions, Serious Illnesses or Accidents

_____

_____

_____

_____

_____

_____

_____

_____

_____

_____

Continue general health information from childhood

_____

_____

_____

_____

_____

_____

_____

_____

_____

_____

_____

_____

_____

_____

_____

_____

_____

_____

_____

_____

_____

_____

_____

Immunizations

Immunization	Date	Reactions? Tolerance?

Vaccinations

Immunization	Date	Reactions? Tolerance?

Pre-Existing Conditions

Condition _____

Diagnosed by Dr._____ Date_____

Experiences with condition and general notes

_____

_____

_____

_____

_____

_____

_____

Condition _____

Diagnosed by Dr._____ Date_____

Experiences with condition and general notes

_____

_____

_____

_____

_____

_____

_____

Pre-Existing Conditions

Condition _____

Diagnosed by Dr. _____ Date_____

Experiences with condition and general notes

_____

_____

_____

_____

_____

_____

_____

Condition _____

Diagnosed by Dr. _____ Date_____

Experiences with condition and general notes

_____

_____

_____

_____

_____

_____

_____

Pre-Existing Conditions

Condition _____

Diagnosed by Dr. _____ Date _____

Experiences with condition and general notes

_____

_____

_____

_____

_____

_____

_____

Condition _____

Diagnosed by Dr. _____ Date _____

Experiences with condition and general notes

_____

_____

_____

_____

_____

_____

_____

_____

Pre-Existing Conditions

Condition _____

Diagnosed by Dr._____ Date_____

Experiences with condition and general notes

_____

_____

_____

_____

_____

_____

_____

Condition _____

Diagnosed by Dr._____ Date_____

Experiences with condition and general notes

_____

_____

_____

_____

_____

_____

_____

General Doctor Visits

The earliest written record that mentions the practice of medicine is Hammurabi's Code from the 18th century BC in Mesopotamia. This extensive code of laws includes information for physicians about payments for successful treatments and punishments for medical failures. For example, payment was better for curing the wealthy, but failing to do so could result in the loss of a hand. https://www.factretriever.com/doctor-facts

Date of Appointment _____ Time_____

Doctor's Name _____ Ph#_____

Address_____

Reason for Visit _____

Diagnosis & Treatment _____

Drugs prescribed _____

List drugs alphabetically in the drug section along with reactions and whether or not the drug was successful in curing the problem.

Date of Appointment _____ Time_____

Doctor's Name _____ Ph#_____

Address_____

Reason for Visit _____

Diagnosis & Treatment _____

Drugs prescribed _____

List drugs alphabetically in the drug section along with reactions and whether or not the drug was successful in curing the problem.

Date of Appointment _____ Time_____

Doctor's Name _____ Ph#_____

Address_____

Reason for Visit _____

Diagnosis & Treatment _____

Drugs prescribed _____

List drugs alphabetically in the drug section along with reactions and whether or not the drug was successful in curing the problem.

Date of Appointment _____ Time_____

Doctor's Name _____ Ph#_____

Address_____

Reason for Visit _____

Diagnosis & Treatment _____

Drugs prescribed _____

List drugs alphabetically in the drug section along with reactions and whether or not the drug was successful in curing the problem.

Date of Appointment _____ Time_____

Doctor's Name _____ Ph#_____

Address_____

Reason for Visit _____

Diagnosis & Treatment _____

Drugs prescribed _____

List drugs alphabetically in the drug section along with reactions and whether or not the drug was successful in curing the problem.

Date of Appointment _____ Time_____

Doctor's Name _____ Ph#_____

Address_____

Reason for Visit _____

Diagnosis & Treatment _____

Drugs prescribed _____

List drugs alphabetically in the drug section along with reactions and whether or not the drug was successful in curing the problem.

Date of Appointment _____ Time_____

Doctor's Name _____ Ph#_____

Address_____

Reason for Visit _____

Diagnosis & Treatment _____

Drugs prescribed _____

List drugs alphabetically in the drug section along with reactions
and whether or not the drug was successful in curing the problem.

Date of Appointment _____ Time_____

Doctor's Name _____ Ph#_____

Address_____

Reason for Visit _____

Diagnosis & Treatment _____

Drugs prescribed _____

List drugs alphabetically in the drug section along with reactions
and whether or not the drug was successful in curing the problem.

Date of Appointment _____ Time_____

Doctor's Name _____ Ph#_____

Address_____

Reason for Visit _____

Diagnosis & Treatment _____

Drugs prescribed _____

List drugs alphabetically in the drug section along with reactions and whether or not the drug was successful in curing the problem.

Date of Appointment _____ Time_____

Doctor's Name _____ Ph#_____

Address_____

Reason for Visit _____

Diagnosis & Treatment _____

Drugs prescribed _____

List drugs alphabetically in the drug section along with reactions and whether or not the drug was successful in curing the problem.

Date of Appointment _____ Time_____

Doctor's Name _____ Ph#_____

Address_____

Reason for Visit _____

Diagnosis & Treatment _____

Drugs prescribed _____

List drugs alphabetically in the drug section along with reactions and whether or not the drug was successful in curing the problem.

Date of Appointment _____ Time_____

Doctor's Name _____ Ph#_____

Address_____

Reason for Visit _____

Diagnosis & Treatment _____

Drugs prescribed _____

List drugs alphabetically in the drug section along with reactions and whether or not the drug was successful in curing the problem.

Date of Appointment _____ Time_____

Doctor's Name _____ Ph#_____

Address_____

Reason for Visit _____

Diagnosis & Treatment _____

Drugs prescribed _____

List drugs alphabetically in the drug section along with reactions and whether or not the drug was successful in curing the problem.

Date of Appointment _____ Time_____

Doctor's Name _____ Ph#_____

Address_____

Reason for Visit _____

Diagnosis & Treatment _____

Drugs prescribed _____

List drugs alphabetically in the drug section along with reactions and whether or not the drug was successful in curing the problem.

Date of Appointment _____ Time_____

Doctor's Name _____ Ph#_____

Address_____

Reason for Visit _____

Diagnosis & Treatment _____

Drugs prescribed _____

List drugs alphabetically in the drug section along with reactions and whether or not the drug was successful in curing the problem.

Date of Appointment _____ Time_____

Doctor's Name _____ Ph#_____

Address_____

Reason for Visit _____

Diagnosis & Treatment _____

Drugs prescribed _____

List drugs alphabetically in the drug section along with reactions and whether or not the drug was successful in curing the problem.

Date of Appointment _____ Time_____

Doctor's Name _____ Ph#_____

Address_____

Reason for Visit _____

Diagnosis & Treatment _____

Drugs prescribed _____

List drugs alphabetically in the drug section along with reactions and whether or not the drug was successful in curing the problem.

Date of Appointment _____ Time_____

Doctor's Name _____ Ph#_____

Address_____

Reason for Visit _____

Diagnosis & Treatment _____

Drugs prescribed _____

List drugs alphabetically in the drug section along with reactions and whether or not the drug was successful in curing the problem.

Date of Appointment _____ Time_____

Doctor's Name _____ Ph#_____

Address_____

Reason for Visit _____

Diagnosis & Treatment _____

Drugs prescribed _____

List drugs alphabetically in the drug section along with reactions and whether or not the drug was successful in curing the problem.

Date of Appointment _____ Time_____

Doctor's Name _____ Ph#_____

Address_____

Reason for Visit _____

Diagnosis & Treatment _____

Drugs prescribed _____

List drugs alphabetically in the drug section along with reactions and whether or not the drug was successful in curing the problem.

Date of Appointment _____ Time_____

Doctor's Name _____ Ph#_____

Address_____

Reason for Visit _____

Diagnosis & Treatment _____

Drugs prescribed _____

List drugs alphabetically in the drug section along with reactions and whether or not the drug was successful in curing the problem.

Date of Appointment _____ Time_____

Doctor's Name _____ Ph#_____

Address_____

Reason for Visit _____

Diagnosis & Treatment _____

Drugs prescribed _____

List drugs alphabetically in the drug section along with reactions and whether or not the drug was successful in curing the problem.

Date of Appointment _____ Time_____

Doctor's Name _____ Ph#_____

Address_____

Reason for Visit _____

Diagnosis & Treatment _____

Drugs prescribed _____

List drugs alphabetically in the drug section along with reactions and whether or not the drug was successful in curing the problem.

Date of Appointment _____ Time_____

Doctor's Name _____ Ph#_____

Address_____

Reason for Visit _____

Diagnosis & Treatment _____

Drugs prescribed _____

List drugs alphabetically in the drug section along with reactions and whether or not the drug was successful in curing the problem.

Date of Appointment _____ Time_____

Doctor's Name _____ Ph#_____

Address_____

Reason for Visit _____

Diagnosis & Treatment _____

Drugs prescribed _____

List drugs alphabetically in the drug section along with reactions and whether or not the drug was successful in curing the problem.

Date of Appointment _____ Time_____

Doctor's Name _____ Ph#_____

Address_____

Reason for Visit _____

Diagnosis & Treatment _____

Drugs prescribed _____

List drugs alphabetically in the drug section along with reactions and whether or not the drug was successful in curing the problem.

Date of Appointment _____ Time_____

Doctor's Name _____ Ph#_____

Address_____

Reason for Visit _____

Diagnosis & Treatment _____

Drugs prescribed _____

List drugs alphabetically in the drug section along with reactions and whether or not the drug was successful in curing the problem.

Date of Appointment _____ Time_____

Doctor's Name _____ Ph#_____

Address_____

Reason for Visit _____

Diagnosis & Treatment _____

Drugs prescribed _____

List drugs alphabetically in the drug section along with reactions and whether or not the drug was successful in curing the problem.

Date of Appointment _____ Time_____

Doctor's Name _____ Ph#_____

Address_____

Reason for Visit _____

Diagnosis & Treatment _____

Drugs prescribed _____

List drugs alphabetically in the drug section along with reactions and whether or not the drug was successful in curing the problem.

Date of Appointment _____ Time_____

Doctor's Name _____ Ph#_____

Address_____

Reason for Visit _____

Diagnosis & Treatment _____

Drugs prescribed _____

List drugs alphabetically in the drug section along with reactions and whether or not the drug was successful in curing the problem.

Date of Appointment _____ Time_____

Doctor's Name _____ Ph#_____

Address_____

Reason for Visit _____

Diagnosis & Treatment _____

Drugs prescribed _____

List drugs alphabetically in the drug section along with reactions and whether or not the drug was successful in curing the problem.

Date of Appointment _____ Time_____

Doctor's Name _____ Ph#_____

Address_____

Reason for Visit _____

Diagnosis & Treatment _____

Drugs prescribed _____

List drugs alphabetically in the drug section along with reactions and whether or not the drug was successful in curing the problem.

Date of Appointment _____ Time_____

Doctor's Name _____ Ph#_____

Address_____

Reason for Visit _____

Diagnosis & Treatment _____

Drugs prescribed _____

List drugs alphabetically in the drug section along with reactions and whether or not the drug was successful in curing the problem.

Date of Appointment _____ Time_____

Doctor's Name _____ Ph#_____

Address_____

Reason for Visit _____

Diagnosis & Treatment _____

Drugs prescribed _____

List drugs alphabetically in the drug section along with reactions and whether or not the drug was successful in curing the problem.

Date of Appointment _____ Time_____

Doctor's Name _____ Ph#_____

Address_____

Reason for Visit _____

Diagnosis & Treatment _____

Drugs prescribed _____

List drugs alphabetically in the drug section along with reactions and whether or not the drug was successful in curing the problem.

Date of Appointment _____ Time_____

Doctor's Name _____ Ph#_____

Address_____

Reason for Visit _____

Diagnosis & Treatment _____

Drugs prescribed _____

List drugs alphabetically in the drug section along with reactions and whether or not the drug was successful in curing the problem.

Date of Appointment _____ Time_____

Doctor's Name _____ Ph#_____

Address_____

Reason for Visit _____

Diagnosis & Treatment _____

Drugs prescribed _____

List drugs alphabetically in the drug section along with reactions and whether or not the drug was successful in curing the problem.

Date of Appointment _____ Time_____

Doctor's Name _____ Ph#_____

Address_____

Reason for Visit _____

Diagnosis & Treatment _____

Drugs prescribed _____

List drugs alphabetically in the drug section along with reactions and whether or not the drug was successful in curing the problem.

Date of Appointment _____ Time_____

Doctor's Name _____ Ph#_____

Address_____

Reason for Visit _____

Diagnosis & Treatment _____

Drugs prescribed _____

List drugs alphabetically in the drug section along with reactions and whether or not the drug was successful in curing the problem.

Date of Appointment _____ Time_____

Doctor's Name _____ Ph#_____

Address_____

Reason for Visit _____

Diagnosis & Treatment _____

Drugs prescribed _____

List drugs alphabetically in the drug section along with reactions and whether or not the drug was successful in curing the problem.

Date of Appointment _____ Time_____

Doctor's Name _____ Ph#_____

Address_____

Reason for Visit _____
_____

Diagnosis & Treatment _____
_____
_____

Drugs prescribed _____
_____
_____

List drugs alphabetically in the drug section along with reactions and whether or not the drug was successful in curing the problem.

Date of Appointment _____ Time_____

Doctor's Name _____ Ph#_____

Address_____

Reason for Visit _____
_____

Diagnosis & Treatment _____
_____
_____

Drugs prescribed _____
_____
_____

List drugs alphabetically in the drug section along with reactions and whether or not the drug was successful in curing the problem.

Date of Appointment _____ Time_____

Doctor's Name _____ Ph#_____

Address_____

Reason for Visit _____

Diagnosis & Treatment _____

Drugs prescribed _____

List drugs alphabetically in the drug section along with reactions
and whether or not the drug was successful in curing the problem.

Date of Appointment _____ Time_____

Doctor's Name _____ Ph#_____

Address_____

Reason for Visit _____

Diagnosis & Treatment _____

Drugs prescribed _____

List drugs alphabetically in the drug section along with reactions
and whether or not the drug was successful in curing the problem.

Date of Appointment _____ Time_____

Doctor's Name _____ Ph#_____

Address_____

Reason for Visit _____

Diagnosis & Treatment _____

Drugs prescribed _____

List drugs alphabetically in the drug section along with reactions and whether or not the drug was successful in curing the problem.

Date of Appointment _____ Time_____

Doctor's Name _____ Ph#_____

Address_____

Reason for Visit _____

Diagnosis & Treatment _____

Drugs prescribed _____

List drugs alphabetically in the drug section along with reactions and whether or not the drug was successful in curing the problem.

Date of Appointment _____ Time_____

Doctor's Name _____ Ph#_____

Address_____

Reason for Visit _____

Diagnosis & Treatment _____

Drugs prescribed _____

List drugs alphabetically in the drug section along with reactions and whether or not the drug was successful in curing the problem.

Date of Appointment _____ Time_____

Doctor's Name _____ Ph#_____

Address_____

Reason for Visit _____

Diagnosis & Treatment _____

Drugs prescribed _____

List drugs alphabetically in the drug section along with reactions and whether or not the drug was successful in curing the problem.

Date of Appointment _____ Time_____

Doctor's Name _____ Ph#_____

Address_____

Reason for Visit _____

Diagnosis & Treatment _____

Drugs prescribed _____

List drugs alphabetically in the drug section along with reactions and whether or not the drug was successful in curing the problem.

Date of Appointment _____ Time_____

Doctor's Name _____ Ph#_____

Address_____

Reason for Visit _____

Diagnosis & Treatment _____

Drugs prescribed _____

List drugs alphabetically in the drug section along with reactions and whether or not the drug was successful in curing the problem.

Date of Appointment _____ Time_____

Doctor's Name _____ Ph#_____

Address_____

Reason for Visit _____

Diagnosis & Treatment _____

Drugs prescribed _____

List drugs alphabetically in the drug section along with reactions and whether or not the drug was successful in curing the problem.

Date of Appointment _____ Time_____

Doctor's Name _____ Ph#_____

Address_____

Reason for Visit _____

Diagnosis & Treatment _____

Drugs prescribed _____

List drugs alphabetically in the drug section along with reactions and whether or not the drug was successful in curing the problem.

Date of Appointment _____ Time_____

Doctor's Name _____ Ph#_____

Address_____

Reason for Visit _____

Diagnosis & Treatment _____

Drugs prescribed _____

List drugs alphabetically in the drug section along with reactions and whether or not the drug was successful in curing the problem.

Date of Appointment _____ Time_____

Doctor's Name _____ Ph#_____

Address_____

Reason for Visit _____

Diagnosis & Treatment _____

Drugs prescribed _____

List drugs alphabetically in the drug section along with reactions and whether or not the drug was successful in curing the problem.

Date of Appointment _____ Time_____

Doctor's Name _____ Ph#_____

Address_____

Reason for Visit _____

Diagnosis & Treatment _____

Drugs prescribed _____

List drugs alphabetically in the drug section along with reactions
and whether or not the drug was successful in curing the problem.

Date of Appointment _____ Time_____

Doctor's Name _____ Ph#_____

Address_____

Reason for Visit _____

Diagnosis & Treatment _____

Drugs prescribed _____

List drugs alphabetically in the drug section along with reactions
and whether or not the drug was successful in curing the problem.

Date of Appointment _____ Time_____

Doctor's Name _____ Ph#_____

Address_____

Reason for Visit _____

Diagnosis & Treatment _____

Drugs prescribed _____

List drugs alphabetically in the drug section along with reactions and whether or not the drug was successful in curing the problem.

Date of Appointment _____ Time_____

Doctor's Name _____ Ph#_____

Address_____

Reason for Visit _____

Diagnosis & Treatment _____

Drugs prescribed _____

List drugs alphabetically in the drug section along with reactions and whether or not the drug was successful in curing the problem.

Date of Appointment _____ Time_____

Doctor's Name _____ Ph#_____

Address_____

Reason for Visit _____

Diagnosis & Treatment _____

Drugs prescribed _____

List drugs alphabetically in the drug section along with reactions
and whether or not the drug was successful in curing the problem.

Date of Appointment _____ Time_____

Doctor's Name _____ Ph#_____

Address_____

Reason for Visit _____

Diagnosis & Treatment _____

Drugs prescribed _____

List drugs alphabetically in the drug section along with reactions
and whether or not the drug was successful in curing the problem.

Date of Appointment _____ Time_____

Doctor's Name _____ Ph#_____

Address_____

Reason for Visit _____

Diagnosis & Treatment _____

Drugs prescribed _____

List drugs alphabetically in the drug section along with reactions and whether or not the drug was successful in curing the problem.

Date of Appointment _____ Time_____

Doctor's Name _____ Ph#_____

Address_____

Reason for Visit _____

Diagnosis & Treatment _____

Drugs prescribed _____

List drugs alphabetically in the drug section along with reactions and whether or not the drug was successful in curing the problem.

Date of Appointment _____ Time_____

Doctor's Name _____ Ph#_____

Address_____

Reason for Visit _____

Diagnosis & Treatment _____

Drugs prescribed _____

List drugs alphabetically in the drug section along with reactions and whether or not the drug was successful in curing the problem.

Date of Appointment _____ Time_____

Doctor's Name _____ Ph#_____

Address_____

Reason for Visit _____

Diagnosis & Treatment _____

Drugs prescribed _____

List drugs alphabetically in the drug section along with reactions and whether or not the drug was successful in curing the problem.

Date of Appointment _____ Time_____

Doctor's Name _____ Ph#_____

Address_____

Reason for Visit _____

Diagnosis & Treatment _____

Drugs prescribed _____

List drugs alphabetically in the drug section along with reactions and whether or not the drug was successful in curing the problem.

Date of Appointment _____ Time_____

Doctor's Name _____ Ph#_____

Address_____

Reason for Visit _____

Diagnosis & Treatment _____

Drugs prescribed _____

List drugs alphabetically in the drug section along with reactions and whether or not the drug was successful in curing the problem.

Date of Appointment _____ Time_____

Doctor's Name _____ Ph#_____

Address_____

Reason for Visit _____

Diagnosis & Treatment _____

Drugs prescribed _____

List drugs alphabetically in the drug section along with reactions
and whether or not the drug was successful in curing the problem.

Date of Appointment _____ Time_____

Doctor's Name _____ Ph#_____

Address_____

Reason for Visit _____

Diagnosis & Treatment _____

Drugs prescribed _____

List drugs alphabetically in the drug section along with reactions
and whether or not the drug was successful in curing the problem.

Date of Appointment _____ Time_____

Doctor's Name _____ Ph#_____

Address_____

Reason for Visit _____

Diagnosis & Treatment _____

Drugs prescribed _____

List drugs alphabetically in the drug section along with reactions and whether or not the drug was successful in curing the problem.

Date of Appointment _____ Time_____

Doctor's Name _____ Ph#_____

Address_____

Reason for Visit _____

Diagnosis & Treatment _____

Drugs prescribed _____

List drugs alphabetically in the drug section along with reactions and whether or not the drug was successful in curing the problem.

Date of Appointment _____ Time_____

Doctor's Name _____ Ph#_____

Address_____

Reason for Visit _____

Diagnosis & Treatment _____

Drugs prescribed _____

List drugs alphabetically in the drug section along with reactions
and whether or not the drug was successful in curing the problem.

Date of Appointment _____ Time_____

Doctor's Name _____ Ph#_____

Address_____

Reason for Visit _____

Diagnosis & Treatment _____

Drugs prescribed _____

List drugs alphabetically in the drug section along with reactions
and whether or not the drug was successful in curing the problem.

Date of Appointment _____ Time_____

Doctor's Name _____ Ph#_____

Address_____

Reason for Visit _____

Diagnosis & Treatment _____

Drugs prescribed _____

List drugs alphabetically in the drug section along with reactions and whether or not the drug was successful in curing the problem.

Date of Appointment _____ Time_____

Doctor's Name _____ Ph#_____

Address_____

Reason for Visit _____

Diagnosis & Treatment _____

Drugs prescribed _____

List drugs alphabetically in the drug section along with reactions and whether or not the drug was successful in curing the problem.

Date of Appointment _____ Time_____

Doctor's Name _____ Ph#_____

Address_____

Reason for Visit _____

Diagnosis & Treatment _____

Drugs prescribed _____

List drugs alphabetically in the drug section along with reactions and whether or not the drug was successful in curing the problem.

Date of Appointment _____ Time_____

Doctor's Name _____ Ph#_____

Address_____

Reason for Visit _____

Diagnosis & Treatment _____

Drugs prescribed _____

List drugs alphabetically in the drug section along with reactions and whether or not the drug was successful in curing the problem.

Date of Appointment _____ Time_____

Doctor's Name _____ Ph#_____

Address_____

Reason for Visit _____

Diagnosis & Treatment _____

Drugs prescribed _____

List drugs alphabetically in the drug section along with reactions and whether or not the drug was successful in curing the problem.

Date of Appointment _____ Time_____

Doctor's Name _____ Ph#_____

Address_____

Reason for Visit _____

Diagnosis & Treatment _____

Drugs prescribed _____

List drugs alphabetically in the drug section along with reactions and whether or not the drug was successful in curing the problem.

Date of Appointment _____ Time_____

Doctor's Name _____ Ph#_____

Address_____

Reason for Visit _____

Diagnosis & Treatment _____

Drugs prescribed _____

List drugs alphabetically in the drug section along with reactions and whether or not the drug was successful in curing the problem.

Date of Appointment _____ Time_____

Doctor's Name _____ Ph#_____

Address_____

Reason for Visit _____

Diagnosis & Treatment _____

Drugs prescribed _____

List drugs alphabetically in the drug section along with reactions and whether or not the drug was successful in curing the problem.

Date of Appointment _____ Time_____

Doctor's Name _____ Ph#_____

Address_____

Reason for Visit _____

Diagnosis & Treatment _____

Drugs prescribed _____

List drugs alphabetically in the drug section along with reactions and whether or not the drug was successful in curing the problem.

Date of Appointment _____ Time_____

Doctor's Name _____ Ph#_____

Address_____

Reason for Visit _____

Diagnosis & Treatment _____

Drugs prescribed _____

List drugs alphabetically in the drug section along with reactions and whether or not the drug was successful in curing the problem.

Date of Appointment _____ Time_____

Doctor's Name _____ Ph#_____

Address_____

Reason for Visit _____

Diagnosis & Treatment _____

Drugs prescribed _____

List drugs alphabetically in the drug section along with reactions and whether or not the drug was successful in curing the problem.

Date of Appointment _____ Time_____

Doctor's Name _____ Ph#_____

Address_____

Reason for Visit _____

Diagnosis & Treatment _____

Drugs prescribed _____

List drugs alphabetically in the drug section along with reactions and whether or not the drug was successful in curing the problem.

Date of Appointment _____ Time_____

Doctor's Name _____ Ph#_____

Address_____

Reason for Visit _____

Diagnosis & Treatment _____

Drugs prescribed _____

List drugs alphabetically in the drug section along with reactions and whether or not the drug was successful in curing the problem.

Date of Appointment _____ Time_____

Doctor's Name _____ Ph#_____

Address_____

Reason for Visit _____

Diagnosis & Treatment _____

Drugs prescribed _____

List drugs alphabetically in the drug section along with reactions and whether or not the drug was successful in curing the problem.

Date of Appointment _____ Time_____

Doctor's Name _____ Ph#_____

Address_____

Reason for Visit _____

Diagnosis & Treatment _____

Drugs prescribed _____

List drugs alphabetically in the drug section along with reactions and whether or not the drug was successful in curing the problem.

Date of Appointment _____ Time_____

Doctor's Name _____ Ph#_____

Address_____

Reason for Visit _____

Diagnosis & Treatment _____

Drugs prescribed _____

List drugs alphabetically in the drug section along with reactions and whether or not the drug was successful in curing the problem.

Date of Appointment _____ Time_____

Doctor's Name _____ Ph#_____

Address_____

Reason for Visit _____

Diagnosis & Treatment _____

Drugs prescribed _____

List drugs alphabetically in the drug section along with reactions and whether or not the drug was successful in curing the problem.

Date of Appointment _____ Time_____

Doctor's Name _____ Ph#_____

Address_____

Reason for Visit _____

Diagnosis & Treatment _____

Drugs prescribed _____

List drugs alphabetically in the drug section along with reactions and whether or not the drug was successful in curing the problem.

Date of Appointment _____ Time_____

Doctor's Name _____ Ph#_____

Address_____

Reason for Visit _____

Diagnosis & Treatment _____

Drugs prescribed _____

List drugs alphabetically in the drug section along with reactions and whether or not the drug was successful in curing the problem.

Date of Appointment _____ Time_____

Doctor's Name _____ Ph#_____

Address_____

Reason for Visit _____

Diagnosis & Treatment _____

Drugs prescribed _____

List drugs alphabetically in the drug section along with reactions and whether or not the drug was successful in curing the problem.

Date of Appointment _____ Time_____

Doctor's Name _____ Ph#_____

Address_____

Reason for Visit _____

Diagnosis & Treatment _____

Drugs prescribed _____

List drugs alphabetically in the drug section along with reactions
and whether or not the drug was successful in curing the problem.

Date of Appointment _____ Time_____

Doctor's Name _____ Ph#_____

Address_____

Reason for Visit _____

Diagnosis & Treatment _____

Drugs prescribed _____

List drugs alphabetically in the drug section along with reactions
and whether or not the drug was successful in curing the problem.

Date of Appointment _____ Time_____

Doctor's Name _____ Ph#_____

Address_____

Reason for Visit _____

Diagnosis & Treatment _____

Drugs prescribed _____

List drugs alphabetically in the drug section along with reactions and whether or not the drug was successful in curing the problem.

Date of Appointment _____ Time_____

Doctor's Name _____ Ph#_____

Address_____

Reason for Visit _____

Diagnosis & Treatment _____

Drugs prescribed _____

List drugs alphabetically in the drug section along with reactions and whether or not the drug was successful in curing the problem.

Date of Appointment _____ Time_____

Doctor's Name _____ Ph#_____

Address_____

Reason for Visit _____

Diagnosis & Treatment _____

Drugs prescribed _____

List drugs alphabetically in the drug section along with reactions and whether or not the drug was successful in curing the problem.

Date of Appointment _____ Time_____

Doctor's Name _____ Ph#_____

Address_____

Reason for Visit _____

Diagnosis & Treatment _____

Drugs prescribed _____

List drugs alphabetically in the drug section along with reactions and whether or not the drug was successful in curing the problem.

Date of Appointment _____ Time_____

Doctor's Name _____ Ph#_____

Address_____

Reason for Visit _____

Diagnosis & Treatment _____

Drugs prescribed _____

List drugs alphabetically in the drug section along with reactions and whether or not the drug was successful in curing the problem.

Date of Appointment _____ Time_____

Doctor's Name _____ Ph#_____

Address_____

Reason for Visit _____

Diagnosis & Treatment _____

Drugs prescribed _____

List drugs alphabetically in the drug section along with reactions and whether or not the drug was successful in curing the problem.

ILLNESS RECORD

List all your illnesses for easy access of recent maladies. Each illness should be referenced back to the Doctor's visit when it was diagnosed.

Illness _____ Date_____
Diagnosed during Doctor's Visit on page _____

Illness _____ Date_____
Diagnosed during Doctor's Visit on page _____

Illness _____ Date_____
Diagnosed during Doctor's Visit on page _____

Illness _____ Date_____
Diagnosed during Doctor's Visit on page _____

Illness _____ Date_____
Diagnosed during Doctor's Visit on page _____

Illness _____ Date_____
Diagnosed during Doctor's Visit on page _____

Illness _____ Date_____
Diagnosed during Doctor's Visit on page _____

Illness _____ Date_____
Diagnosed during Doctor's Visit on page _____

Illness _____ Date_____
Diagnosed during Doctor's Visit on page _____

Illness _____ Date_____

Diagnosed during Doctor's Visit on page _____

Illness _____ Date_____

Diagnosed during Doctor's Visit on page _____

Illness _____ Date_____

Diagnosed during Doctor's Visit on page _____

Illness _____ Date_____

Diagnosed during Doctor's Visit on page _____

Illness _____ Date_____

Diagnosed during Doctor's Visit on page _____

Illness _____ Date_____

Diagnosed during Doctor's Visit on page _____

Illness _____ Date_____

Diagnosed during Doctor's Visit on page _____

Illness _____ Date_____

Diagnosed during Doctor's Visit on page _____

Illness _____ Date_____

Diagnosed during Doctor's Visit on page _____

Illness _____ Date_____

Diagnosed during Doctor's Visit on page _____

Illness _____ Date_____

Diagnosed during Doctor's Visit on page _____

Illness _____ Date_____

Diagnosed during Doctor's Visit on page _____

Illness _____ Date_____

Diagnosed during Doctor's Visit on page _____

Illness _____ Date_____

Diagnosed during Doctor's Visit on page _____

Illness _____ Date_____

Diagnosed during Doctor's Visit on page _____

Illness _____ Date_____

Diagnosed during Doctor's Visit on page _____

Illness _____ Date_____

Diagnosed during Doctor's Visit on page _____

Illness _____ Date_____

Diagnosed during Doctor's Visit on page _____

Illness _____ Date_____

Diagnosed during Doctor's Visit on page _____

Illness _____ Date_____

Diagnosed during Doctor's Visit on page _____

Illness _____ Date_____

Diagnosed during Doctor's Visit on page _____

Illness _____ Date_____

Diagnosed during Doctor's Visit on page _____

Illness _____ Date_____
Diagnosed during Doctor's Visit on page _____

Illness _____ Date_____
Diagnosed during Doctor's Visit on page _____

Illness _____ Date_____
Diagnosed during Doctor's Visit on page _____

Illness _____ Date_____
Diagnosed during Doctor's Visit on page _____

Illness _____ Date_____
Diagnosed during Doctor's Visit on page _____

Illness _____ Date_____
Diagnosed during Doctor's Visit on page _____

Illness _____ Date_____
Diagnosed during Doctor's Visit on page _____

Illness _____ Date_____
Diagnosed during Doctor's Visit on page _____

Illness _____ Date_____
Diagnosed during Doctor's Visit on page _____

Illness _____ Date_____
Diagnosed during Doctor's Visit on page _____

Illness _____ Date_____
Diagnosed during Doctor's Visit on page _____

Doctor Visits
Specialty

This section is for Specialty Doctor's appointments: Cardiologist, Internists, Urologist, Orthopedists etc.

What is the oldest medical specialty?

Otolaryngology

Doctors developed techniques and tools for examining and treating problems of the head and neck, eventually forming a medical specialty. According to the American Academy of **Otolaryngology**, it is the oldest medical specialty in the United States.

Specialty_____ Date_____ Time _____

Doctor's Name _____ Ph#_____

Address_____

Reason for Visit _____

Diagnosis & Treatment _____

Drugs prescribed _____

List drugs alphabetically in the drug section along with reactions and whether or not the drug was successful in curing the problem.

Specialty_____ Date_____ Time _____

Doctor's Name _____ Ph#_____

Address_____

Reason for Visit _____

Diagnosis & Treatment _____

Drugs prescribed _____

List drugs alphabetically in the drug section along with reactions and whether or not the drug was successful in curing the problem.

Specialty_____ Date_____ Time _____

Doctor's Name _____ Ph#_____

Address_____

Reason for Visit _____

Diagnosis & Treatment _____

Drugs prescribed _____

List drugs alphabetically in the drug section along with reactions and whether or not the drug was successful in curing the problem.

Specialty_____ Date_____ Time _____

Doctor's Name _____ Ph#_____

Address_____

Reason for Visit _____

Diagnosis & Treatment _____

Drugs prescribed _____

List drugs alphabetically in the drug section along with reactions and whether or not the drug was successful in curing the problem.

Specialty_____ Date_____ Time _____

Doctor's Name _____ Ph#_____

Address_____

Reason for Visit _____

Diagnosis & Treatment _____

Drugs prescribed _____

List drugs alphabetically in the drug section along with reactions and whether or not the drug was successful in curing the problem.

Specialty_____ Date_____ Time _____

Doctor's Name _____ Ph#_____

Address_____

Reason for Visit _____

Diagnosis & Treatment _____

Drugs prescribed _____

List drugs alphabetically in the drug section along with reactions and whether or not the drug was successful in curing the problem.

Specialty_____ Date_____ Time _____

Doctor's Name _____ Ph#_____

Address_____

Reason for Visit _____

Diagnosis & Treatment _____

Drugs prescribed _____

List drugs alphabetically in the drug section along with reactions and whether or not the drug was successful in curing the problem.

Specialty_____ Date_____ Time _____

Doctor's Name _____ Ph#_____

Address_____

Reason for Visit _____

Diagnosis & Treatment _____

Drugs prescribed _____

List drugs alphabetically in the drug section along with reactions and whether or not the drug was successful in curing the problem.

Specialty_____ Date_____ Time _____

Doctor's Name _____ Ph#_____

Address_____

Reason for Visit _____

Diagnosis & Treatment _____

Drugs prescribed _____

List drugs alphabetically in the drug section along with reactions and whether or not the drug was successful in curing the problem.

Specialty_____ Date_____ Time _____

Doctor's Name _____ Ph#_____

Address_____

Reason for Visit _____

Diagnosis & Treatment _____

Drugs prescribed _____

List drugs alphabetically in the drug section along with reactions and whether or not the drug was successful in curing the problem.

Specialty_____ Date_____ Time _____

Doctor's Name _____ Ph#_____

Address_____

Reason for Visit _____

Diagnosis & Treatment _____

Drugs prescribed _____

List drugs alphabetically in the drug section along with reactions and whether or not the drug was successful in curing the problem.

Specialty_____ Date_____ Time _____

Doctor's Name _____ Ph#_____

Address_____

Reason for Visit _____

Diagnosis & Treatment _____

Drugs prescribed _____

List drugs alphabetically in the drug section along with reactions and whether or not the drug was successful in curing the problem.

Specialty_____ Date_____ Time _____

Doctor's Name _____ Ph#_____

Address_____

Reason for Visit _____

Diagnosis & Treatment _____

Drugs prescribed _____

List drugs alphabetically in the drug section along with reactions and whether or not the drug was successful in curing the problem.

Specialty_____ Date_____ Time _____

Doctor's Name _____ Ph#_____

Address_____

Reason for Visit _____

Diagnosis & Treatment _____

Drugs prescribed _____

List drugs alphabetically in the drug section along with reactions and whether or not the drug was successful in curing the problem.

Specialty_____ Date_____ Time _____

Doctor's Name _____ Ph#_____

Address_____

Reason for Visit _____

Diagnosis & Treatment _____

_____

_____

Drugs prescribed _____

_____

List drugs alphabetically in the drug section along with reactions and whether or not the drug was successful in curing the problem.

Specialty_____ Date_____ Time _____

Doctor's Name _____ Ph#_____

Address_____

Reason for Visit _____

Diagnosis & Treatment _____

_____

_____

Drugs prescribed _____

_____

List drugs alphabetically in the drug section along with reactions and whether or not the drug was successful in curing the problem.

Specialty_____ Date_____ Time _____

Doctor's Name _____ Ph#_____

Address_____

Reason for Visit _____

Diagnosis & Treatment _____

_____

_____

Drugs prescribed _____

_____

List drugs alphabetically in the drug section along with reactions and whether or not the drug was successful in curing the problem.

Specialty_____ Date_____ Time _____

Doctor's Name _____ Ph#_____

Address_____

Reason for Visit _____

Diagnosis & Treatment _____

_____

_____

Drugs prescribed _____

_____

List drugs alphabetically in the drug section along with reactions and whether or not the drug was successful in curing the problem.

Specialty_____ Date_____ Time _____

Doctor's Name _____ Ph#_____

Address_____

Reason for Visit _____

Diagnosis & Treatment _____

Drugs prescribed _____

List drugs alphabetically in the drug section along with reactions
and whether or not the drug was successful in curing the problem.

Specialty_____ Date_____ Time _____

Doctor's Name _____ Ph#_____

Address_____

Reason for Visit _____

Diagnosis & Treatment _____

Drugs prescribed _____

List drugs alphabetically in the drug section along with reactions
and whether or not the drug was successful in curing the problem.

Specialty_____ Date_____ Time _____

Doctor's Name _____ Ph#_____

Address_____

Reason for Visit _____

Diagnosis & Treatment _____

_____

_____

Drugs prescribed _____

_____

List drugs alphabetically in the drug section along with reactions and whether or not the drug was successful in curing the problem.

Specialty_____ Date_____ Time _____

Doctor's Name _____ Ph#_____

Address_____

Reason for Visit _____

Diagnosis & Treatment _____

_____

_____

Drugs prescribed _____

_____

List drugs alphabetically in the drug section along with reactions and whether or not the drug was successful in curing the problem.

Specialty_____ Date_____ Time _____

Doctor's Name _____ Ph#_____

Address_____

Reason for Visit _____

Diagnosis & Treatment _____

Drugs prescribed _____

List drugs alphabetically in the drug section along with reactions and whether or not the drug was successful in curing the problem.

Specialty_____ Date_____ Time _____

Doctor's Name _____ Ph#_____

Address_____

Reason for Visit _____

Diagnosis & Treatment _____

Drugs prescribed _____

List drugs alphabetically in the drug section along with reactions and whether or not the drug was successful in curing the problem.

Specialty_____ Date_____ Time _____

Doctor's Name _____ Ph#_____

Address_____

Reason for Visit _____

Diagnosis & Treatment _____

Drugs prescribed _____

List drugs alphabetically in the drug section along with reactions and whether or not the drug was successful in curing the problem.

Specialty_____ Date_____ Time _____

Doctor's Name _____ Ph#_____

Address_____

Reason for Visit _____

Diagnosis & Treatment _____

Drugs prescribed _____

List drugs alphabetically in the drug section along with reactions and whether or not the drug was successful in curing the problem.

Specialty_____ Date_____ Time _____

Doctor's Name _____ Ph#_____

Address_____

Reason for Visit _____

Diagnosis & Treatment _____

Drugs prescribed _____

List drugs alphabetically in the drug section along with reactions and whether or not the drug was successful in curing the problem.

Specialty_____ Date_____ Time _____

Doctor's Name _____ Ph#_____

Address_____

Reason for Visit _____

Diagnosis & Treatment _____

Drugs prescribed _____

List drugs alphabetically in the drug section along with reactions and whether or not the drug was successful in curing the problem.

Specialty_____ Date_____ Time _____

Doctor's Name _____ Ph#_____

Address_____

Reason for Visit _____

Diagnosis & Treatment _____

Drugs prescribed _____

List drugs alphabetically in the drug section along with reactions and whether or not the drug was successful in curing the problem.

Specialty_____ Date_____ Time _____

Doctor's Name _____ Ph#_____

Address_____

Reason for Visit _____

Diagnosis & Treatment _____

Drugs prescribed _____

List drugs alphabetically in the drug section along with reactions and whether or not the drug was successful in curing the problem.

Specialty_____ Date_____ Time _____

Doctor's Name _____ Ph#_____

Address_____

Reason for Visit _____

Diagnosis & Treatment _____

Drugs prescribed _____

List drugs alphabetically in the drug section along with reactions and whether or not the drug was successful in curing the problem.

Specialty_____ Date_____ Time _____

Doctor's Name _____ Ph#_____

Address_____

Reason for Visit _____

Diagnosis & Treatment _____

Drugs prescribed _____

List drugs alphabetically in the drug section along with reactions and whether or not the drug was successful in curing the problem.

Specialty_____ Date_____ Time _____

Doctor's Name _____ Ph#_____

Address_____

Reason for Visit _____

Diagnosis & Treatment _____

Drugs prescribed _____

List drugs alphabetically in the drug section along with reactions and whether or not the drug was successful in curing the problem.

Specialty_____ Date_____ Time _____

Doctor's Name _____ Ph#_____

Address_____

Reason for Visit _____

Diagnosis & Treatment _____

Drugs prescribed _____

List drugs alphabetically in the drug section along with reactions and whether or not the drug was successful in curing the problem.

Specialty_____ Date_____ Time _____

Doctor's Name _____ Ph#_____

Address_____

Reason for Visit _____

Diagnosis & Treatment _____

Drugs prescribed _____

List drugs alphabetically in the drug section along with reactions and whether or not the drug was successful in curing the problem.

Specialty_____ Date_____ Time _____

Doctor's Name _____ Ph#_____

Address_____

Reason for Visit _____

Diagnosis & Treatment _____

Drugs prescribed _____

List drugs alphabetically in the drug section along with reactions and whether or not the drug was successful in curing the problem.

Specialty_____ Date_____ Time _____

Doctor's Name _____ Ph#_____

Address_____

Reason for Visit _____

Diagnosis & Treatment _____

Drugs prescribed _____

List drugs alphabetically in the drug section along with reactions and whether or not the drug was successful in curing the problem.

Specialty_____ Date_____ Time _____

Doctor's Name _____ Ph#_____

Address_____

Reason for Visit _____

Diagnosis & Treatment _____

Drugs prescribed _____

List drugs alphabetically in the drug section along with reactions and whether or not the drug was successful in curing the problem.

Specialty_____ Date_____ Time _____

Doctor's Name _____ Ph#_____

Address_____

Reason for Visit _____

Diagnosis & Treatment _____

Drugs prescribed _____

List drugs alphabetically in the drug section along with reactions and whether or not the drug was successful in curing the problem.

Specialty_____ Date_____ Time _____

Doctor's Name _____ Ph#_____

Address_____

Reason for Visit _____

Diagnosis & Treatment _____

Drugs prescribed _____

List drugs alphabetically in the drug section along with reactions and whether or not the drug was successful in curing the problem.

Specialty_____ Date_____ Time _____

Doctor's Name _____ Ph#_____

Address_____

Reason for Visit _____

Diagnosis & Treatment _____

_____

Drugs prescribed _____

_____

List drugs alphabetically in the drug section along with reactions and whether or not the drug was successful in curing the problem.

Specialty_____ Date_____ Time _____

Doctor's Name _____ Ph#_____

Address_____

Reason for Visit _____

Diagnosis & Treatment _____

_____

Drugs prescribed _____

_____

List drugs alphabetically in the drug section along with reactions and whether or not the drug was successful in curing the problem.

Specialty_____ Date_____ Time _____

Doctor's Name _____ Ph#_____

Address_____

Reason for Visit _____

Diagnosis & Treatment _____

Drugs prescribed _____

List drugs alphabetically in the drug section along with reactions and whether or not the drug was successful in curing the problem.

Specialty_____ Date_____ Time _____

Doctor's Name _____ Ph#_____

Address_____

Reason for Visit _____

Diagnosis & Treatment _____

Drugs prescribed _____

List drugs alphabetically in the drug section along with reactions and whether or not the drug was successful in curing the problem.

Specialty_____ Date_____ Time _____

Doctor's Name _____ Ph#_____

Address_____

Reason for Visit _____

Diagnosis & Treatment _____

Drugs prescribed _____

List drugs alphabetically in the drug section along with reactions and whether or not the drug was successful in curing the problem.

Specialty_____ Date_____ Time _____

Doctor's Name _____ Ph#_____

Address_____

Reason for Visit _____

Diagnosis & Treatment _____

Drugs prescribed _____

List drugs alphabetically in the drug section along with reactions and whether or not the drug was successful in curing the problem.

Specialty_____ Date_____ Time _____

Doctor's Name _____ Ph#_____

Address_____

Reason for Visit _____

Diagnosis & Treatment _____

Drugs prescribed _____

List drugs alphabetically in the drug section along with reactions and whether or not the drug was successful in curing the problem.

Specialty_____ Date_____ Time _____

Doctor's Name _____ Ph#_____

Address_____

Reason for Visit _____

Diagnosis & Treatment _____

Drugs prescribed _____

List drugs alphabetically in the drug section along with reactions and whether or not the drug was successful in curing the problem.

Prescriptions

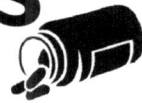

Pharmacies and drugstores have been around for a long time. The world's oldest prescriptions were etched into tablets around 2100 B.C. and Baghdad was home to some of the earliest drugstores, dating as far back as the eighth century. Rxinsider.com

In 1886, pharmacist John S. Pemberton created Coca-Cola as a treatment for most common ailments. His book-keeper, Frank Robinson, names the drink and writes it down in the loopy, flowing handwriting that became known as the brand's logo. The drink was based on co-caine from the coca leaf and caffeinated extracts from a kola nut – hence the name, Coca-Cola. The cocaine was removed from the recipes in 1903. Pemberton sold his syrup to Atlanta soda fountains, and the rest is history. Rxinsider.com

MEDICATION ALLERGIES

Medication Name _____ Date _____
Allergic Reaction _____

Medication Name _____ Date _____
Allergic Reaction _____

Medication Name _____ Date _____
Allergic Reaction _____

Medication Name _____ Date _____
Allergic Reaction _____

Medication Name _____ Date _____
Allergic Reaction _____

Medication Name _____ Date _____
Allergic Reaction _____

Medication Name _____ Date _____
Allergic Reaction _____

Medication Name _____ Date _____
Allergic Reaction _____

Medication Name _____ Date _____
Allergic Reaction _____

Medication Name _____ Date _____
Allergic Reaction _____

Medication Name _____ Date _____
Allergic Reaction _____

CURRENT MEDICATIONS

Use this list for a quick reference of current medications that you are taking. If you stop taking one of these drugs, make an X in the box on the right.

Medication Name	Dosage	Start Date	End Date	X

Medication Name	Dosage	Start Date	End Date	X

A

Date _____

Drug Name _____

Prescribed for: (Flu, pain, etc) _____

Dosage _____ Schedule _____ Pharmacy _____

Did medicine cure the problem? Y N   Would I use it again? Y N

List any side effects _____

This medicine was prescribed during the doctor visit on page _____

Date _____

Drug Name _____

Prescribed for: (Flu, pain, etc) _____

Dosage _____ Schedule _____ Pharmacy _____

Did medicine cure the problem? Y N   Would I use it again? Y N

List any side effects _____

This medicine was prescribed during the doctor visit on page _____

Date _____

Drug Name _____

Prescribed for: (Flu, pain, etc) _____

Dosage _____ Schedule _____ Pharmacy _____

Did medicine cure the problem? Y N   Would I use it again? Y N

List any side effects _____

This medicine was prescribed during the doctor visit on page _____

Date _____

Drug Name _____

Prescribed for: (Flu, pain, etc) _____

Dosage _____ Schedule _____ Pharmacy _____

Did medicine cure the problem? Y N   Would I use it again? Y N

List any side effects _____

This medicine was prescribed during the doctor visit on page _____

Date _____ **A**

Drug Name _____

Prescribed for: (Flu, pain, etc) _____

Dosage _____ Schedule _____ Pharmacy_____

Did medicine cure the problem? Y N   Would I use it again? Y N

List any side effects _____

This medicine was prescribed during the doctor visit on page_____

Date _____

Drug Name _____

Prescribed for: (Flu, pain, etc) _____

Dosage _____ Schedule _____ Pharmacy_____

Did medicine cure the problem? Y N   Would I use it again? Y N

List any side effects _____

This medicine was prescribed during the doctor visit on page_____

Date _____

Drug Name _____

Prescribed for: (Flu, pain, etc) _____

Dosage _____ Schedule _____ Pharmacy_____

Did medicine cure the problem? Y N   Would I use it again? Y N

List any side effects _____

This medicine was prescribed during the doctor visit on page_____

Date _____

Drug Name _____

Prescribed for: (Flu, pain, etc) _____

Dosage _____ Schedule _____ Pharmacy_____

Did medicine cure the problem? Y N   Would I use it again? Y N

List any side effects _____

This medicine was prescribed during the doctor visit on page_____

B

Date

Drug Name _____

Prescribed for: (Flu, pain, etc) _____

Dosage _____ Schedule _____ Pharmacy_____

Did medicine cure the problem? Y N   Would I use it again? Y N

List any side effects _____

This medicine was prescribed during the doctor visit on page____

Date

Drug Name _____

Prescribed for: (Flu, pain, etc) _____

Dosage _____ Schedule _____ Pharmacy_____

Did medicine cure the problem? Y N   Would I use it again? Y N

List any side effects _____

This medicine was prescribed during the doctor visit on page____

Date

Drug Name _____

Prescribed for: (Flu, pain, etc) _____

Dosage _____ Schedule _____ Pharmacy_____

Did medicine cure the problem? Y N   Would I use it again? Y N

List any side effects _____

This medicine was prescribed during the doctor visit on page____

Date

Drug Name _____

Prescribed for: (Flu, pain, etc) _____

Dosage _____ Schedule _____ Pharmacy_____

Did medicine cure the problem? Y N   Would I use it again? Y N

List any side effects _____

This medicine was prescribed during the doctor visit on page____

B

Date _____

Drug Name _____
Prescribed for: (Flu, pain, etc) _____
Dosage _____ Schedule _____ Pharmacy _____
Did medicine cure the problem? Y N   Would I use it again? Y N
List any side effects _____
This medicine was prescribed during the doctor visit on page _____

Date _____

Drug Name _____
Prescribed for: (Flu, pain, etc) _____
Dosage _____ Schedule _____ Pharmacy _____
Did medicine cure the problem? Y N   Would I use it again? Y N
List any side effects _____
This medicine was prescribed during the doctor visit on page _____

Date _____

Drug Name _____
Prescribed for: (Flu, pain, etc) _____
Dosage _____ Schedule _____ Pharmacy _____
Did medicine cure the problem? Y N   Would I use it again? Y N
List any side effects _____
This medicine was prescribed during the doctor visit on page _____

Date _____

Drug Name _____
Prescribed for: (Flu, pain, etc) _____
Dosage _____ Schedule _____ Pharmacy _____
Did medicine cure the problem? Y N   Would I use it again? Y N
List any side effects _____
This medicine was prescribed during the doctor visit on page _____

C

Date _____

Drug Name _____
Prescribed for: (Flu, pain, etc) _____
Dosage _____ Schedule _____ Pharmacy _____
Did medicine cure the problem? Y N   Would I use it again? Y   N
List any side effects _____

This medicine was prescribed during the doctor visit on page _____

Date _____

Drug Name _____
Prescribed for: (Flu, pain, etc) _____
Dosage _____ Schedule _____ Pharmacy _____
Did medicine cure the problem? Y N   Would I use it again? Y   N
List any side effects _____

This medicine was prescribed during the doctor visit on page _____

Date _____

Drug Name _____
Prescribed for: (Flu, pain, etc) _____
Dosage _____ Schedule _____ Pharmacy _____
Did medicine cure the problem? Y N   Would I use it again? Y   N
List any side effects _____

This medicine was prescribed during the doctor visit on page _____

Date _____

Drug Name _____
Prescribed for: (Flu, pain, etc) _____
Dosage _____ Schedule _____ Pharmacy _____
Did medicine cure the problem? Y N   Would I use it again? Y   N
List any side effects _____

This medicine was prescribed during the doctor visit on page _____

Date _____ **C**

Drug Name _____

Prescribed for: (Flu, pain, etc) _____

Dosage _____ Schedule _____ Pharmacy _____

Did medicine cure the problem? Y N   Would I use it again? Y N

List any side effects _____

This medicine was prescribed during the doctor visit on page _____

Date _____

Drug Name _____

Prescribed for: (Flu, pain, etc) _____

Dosage _____ Schedule _____ Pharmacy _____

Did medicine cure the problem? Y N   Would I use it again? Y N

List any side effects _____

This medicine was prescribed during the doctor visit on page _____

Date _____

Drug Name _____

Prescribed for: (Flu, pain, etc) _____

Dosage _____ Schedule _____ Pharmacy _____

Did medicine cure the problem? Y N   Would I use it again? Y N

List any side effects _____

This medicine was prescribed during the doctor visit on page _____

Date _____

Drug Name _____

Prescribed for: (Flu, pain, etc) _____

Dosage _____ Schedule _____ Pharmacy _____

Did medicine cure the problem? Y N   Would I use it again? Y N

List any side effects _____

This medicine was prescribed during the doctor visit on page _____

D

Date

Drug Name _____

Prescribed for: (Flu, pain, etc) _____

Dosage _____ Schedule _____ Pharmacy_____

Did medicine cure the problem? Y N Would I use it again? Y N

List any side effects _____

This medicine was prescribed during the doctor visit on page_____

Date

Drug Name _____

Prescribed for: (Flu, pain, etc) _____

Dosage _____ Schedule _____ Pharmacy_____

Did medicine cure the problem? Y N Would I use it again? Y N

List any side effects _____

This medicine was prescribed during the doctor visit on page_____

Date

Drug Name _____

Prescribed for: (Flu, pain, etc) _____

Dosage _____ Schedule _____ Pharmacy_____

Did medicine cure the problem? Y N Would I use it again? Y N

List any side effects _____

This medicine was prescribed during the doctor visit on page_____

Date

Drug Name _____

Prescribed for: (Flu, pain, etc) _____

Dosage _____ Schedule _____ Pharmacy_____

Did medicine cure the problem? Y N Would I use it again? Y N

List any side effects _____

This medicine was prescribed during the doctor visit on page_____

D

Date _____

Drug Name _____

Prescribed for: (Flu, pain, etc) _____

Dosage _____ Schedule _____ Pharmacy _____

Did medicine cure the problem? Y N   Would I use it again? Y N

List any side effects _____

This medicine was prescribed during the doctor visit on page _____

Date _____

Drug Name _____

Prescribed for: (Flu, pain, etc) _____

Dosage _____ Schedule _____ Pharmacy _____

Did medicine cure the problem? Y N   Would I use it again? Y N

List any side effects _____

This medicine was prescribed during the doctor visit on page _____

Date _____

Drug Name _____

Prescribed for: (Flu, pain, etc) _____

Dosage _____ Schedule _____ Pharmacy _____

Did medicine cure the problem? Y N   Would I use it again? Y N

List any side effects _____

This medicine was prescribed during the doctor visit on page _____

Date _____

Drug Name _____

Prescribed for: (Flu, pain, etc) _____

Dosage _____ Schedule _____ Pharmacy _____

Did medicine cure the problem? Y N   Would I use it again? Y N

List any side effects _____

This medicine was prescribed during the doctor visit on page _____

E

Date _____

Drug Name _____

Prescribed for: (Flu, pain, etc) _____

Dosage _____ Schedule _____ Pharmacy_____

Did medicine cure the problem? Y N Would I use it again? Y N

List any side effects _____

This medicine was prescribed during the doctor visit on page_____

Date _____

Drug Name _____

Prescribed for: (Flu, pain, etc) _____

Dosage _____ Schedule _____ Pharmacy_____

Did medicine cure the problem? Y N Would I use it again? Y N

List any side effects _____

This medicine was prescribed during the doctor visit on page_____

Date _____

Drug Name _____

Prescribed for: (Flu, pain, etc) _____

Dosage _____ Schedule _____ Pharmacy_____

Did medicine cure the problem? Y N Would I use it again? Y N

List any side effects _____

This medicine was prescribed during the doctor visit on page_____

Date _____

Drug Name _____

Prescribed for: (Flu, pain, etc) _____

Dosage _____ Schedule _____ Pharmacy_____

Did medicine cure the problem? Y N Would I use it again? Y N

List any side effects _____

This medicine was prescribed during the doctor visit on page_____

Date _____

Drug Name _____
Prescribed for: (Flu, pain, etc) _____
Dosage _____ Schedule _____ Pharmacy _____
Did medicine cure the problem? Y N   Would I use it again? Y N
List any side effects _____

This medicine was prescribed during the doctor visit on page _____

Date _____

Drug Name _____
Prescribed for: (Flu, pain, etc) _____
Dosage _____ Schedule _____ Pharmacy _____
Did medicine cure the problem? Y N   Would I use it again? Y N
List any side effects _____

This medicine was prescribed during the doctor visit on page _____

Date _____

Drug Name _____
Prescribed for: (Flu, pain, etc) _____
Dosage _____ Schedule _____ Pharmacy _____
Did medicine cure the problem? Y N   Would I use it again? Y N
List any side effects _____

This medicine was prescribed during the doctor visit on page _____

Date _____

Drug Name _____
Prescribed for: (Flu, pain, etc) _____
Dosage _____ Schedule _____ Pharmacy _____
Did medicine cure the problem? Y N   Would I use it again? Y N
List any side effects _____

This medicine was prescribed during the doctor visit on page _____

F

Date _____

Drug Name _____

Prescribed for: (Flu, pain, etc) _____

Dosage _____ Schedule _____ Pharmacy _____

Did medicine cure the problem? Y N Would I use it again? Y N

List any side effects _____

This medicine was prescribed during the doctor visit on page _____

Date _____

Drug Name _____

Prescribed for: (Flu, pain, etc) _____

Dosage _____ Schedule _____ Pharmacy _____

Did medicine cure the problem? Y N Would I use it again? Y N

List any side effects _____

This medicine was prescribed during the doctor visit on page _____

Date _____

Drug Name _____

Prescribed for: (Flu, pain, etc) _____

Dosage _____ Schedule _____ Pharmacy _____

Did medicine cure the problem? Y N Would I use it again? Y N

List any side effects _____

This medicine was prescribed during the doctor visit on page _____

Date _____

Drug Name _____

Prescribed for: (Flu, pain, etc) _____

Dosage _____ Schedule _____ Pharmacy _____

Did medicine cure the problem? Y N Would I use it again? Y N

List any side effects _____

This medicine was prescribed during the doctor visit on page _____

F

Date _____

Drug Name _____

Prescribed for: (Flu, pain, etc) _____

Dosage _____ Schedule _____ Pharmacy_____

Did medicine cure the problem? Y N Would I use it again? Y N

List any side effects _____

This medicine was prescribed during the doctor visit on page____

Date _____

Drug Name _____

Prescribed for: (Flu, pain, etc) _____

Dosage _____ Schedule _____ Pharmacy_____

Did medicine cure the problem? Y N Would I use it again? Y N

List any side effects _____

This medicine was prescribed during the doctor visit on page____

Date _____

Drug Name _____

Prescribed for: (Flu, pain, etc) _____

Dosage _____ Schedule _____ Pharmacy_____

Did medicine cure the problem? Y N Would I use it again? Y N

List any side effects _____

This medicine was prescribed during the doctor visit on page____

Date _____

Drug Name _____

Prescribed for: (Flu, pain, etc) _____

Dosage _____ Schedule _____ Pharmacy_____

Did medicine cure the problem? Y N Would I use it again? Y N

List any side effects _____

This medicine was prescribed during the doctor visit on page____

G

Date _____

Drug Name _____

Prescribed for: (Flu, pain, etc) _____

Dosage _____ Schedule _____ Pharmacy _____

Did medicine cure the problem? Y N Would I use it again? Y N

List any side effects _____

This medicine was prescribed during the doctor visit on page _____

Date _____

Drug Name _____

Prescribed for: (Flu, pain, etc) _____

Dosage _____ Schedule _____ Pharmacy _____

Did medicine cure the problem? Y N Would I use it again? Y N

List any side effects _____

This medicine was prescribed during the doctor visit on page _____

Date _____

Drug Name _____

Prescribed for: (Flu, pain, etc) _____

Dosage _____ Schedule _____ Pharmacy _____

Did medicine cure the problem? Y N Would I use it again? Y N

List any side effects _____

This medicine was prescribed during the doctor visit on page _____

Date _____

Drug Name _____

Prescribed for: (Flu, pain, etc) _____

Dosage _____ Schedule _____ Pharmacy _____

Did medicine cure the problem? Y N Would I use it again? Y N

List any side effects _____

This medicine was prescribed during the doctor visit on page _____

G

Date _____

Drug Name _____

Prescribed for: (Flu, pain, etc) _____

Dosage _____ Schedule _____ Pharmacy _____

Did medicine cure the problem? Y N Would I use it again? Y N

List any side effects _____

This medicine was prescribed during the doctor visit on page _____

Date _____

Drug Name _____

Prescribed for: (Flu, pain, etc) _____

Dosage _____ Schedule _____ Pharmacy _____

Did medicine cure the problem? Y N Would I use it again? Y N

List any side effects _____

This medicine was prescribed during the doctor visit on page _____

Date _____

Drug Name _____

Prescribed for: (Flu, pain, etc) _____

Dosage _____ Schedule _____ Pharmacy _____

Did medicine cure the problem? Y N Would I use it again? Y N

List any side effects _____

This medicine was prescribed during the doctor visit on page _____

Date _____

Drug Name _____

Prescribed for: (Flu, pain, etc) _____

Dosage _____ Schedule _____ Pharmacy _____

Did medicine cure the problem? Y N Would I use it again? Y N

List any side effects _____

This medicine was prescribed during the doctor visit on page _____

H

Date

Drug Name _____

Prescribed for: (Flu, pain, etc) _____

Dosage _____ Schedule _____ Pharmacy_____

Did medicine cure the problem? Y N Would I use it again? Y N

List any side effects _____

This medicine was prescribed during the doctor visit on page_____

Date

Drug Name _____

Prescribed for: (Flu, pain, etc) _____

Dosage _____ Schedule _____ Pharmacy_____

Did medicine cure the problem? Y N Would I use it again? Y N

List any side effects _____

This medicine was prescribed during the doctor visit on page_____

Date

Drug Name _____

Prescribed for: (Flu, pain, etc) _____

Dosage _____ Schedule _____ Pharmacy_____

Did medicine cure the problem? Y N Would I use it again? Y N

List any side effects _____

This medicine was prescribed during the doctor visit on page_____

Date

Drug Name _____

Prescribed for: (Flu, pain, etc) _____

Dosage _____ Schedule _____ Pharmacy_____

Did medicine cure the problem? Y N Would I use it again? Y N

List any side effects _____

This medicine was prescribed during the doctor visit on page_____

Drug Name _____

Prescribed for: (Flu, pain, etc) _____

Dosage _____ Schedule _____ Pharmacy_____

Did medicine cure the problem? Y N Would I use it again? Y N

List any side effects _____

This medicine was prescribed during the doctor visit on page_____

Date

Drug Name _____

Prescribed for: (Flu, pain, etc) _____

Dosage _____ Schedule _____ Pharmacy_____

Did medicine cure the problem? Y N Would I use it again? Y N

List any side effects _____

This medicine was prescribed during the doctor visit on page_____

Date

Drug Name _____

Prescribed for: (Flu, pain, etc) _____

Dosage _____ Schedule _____ Pharmacy_____

Did medicine cure the problem? Y N Would I use it again? Y N

List any side effects _____

This medicine was prescribed during the doctor visit on page_____

Date

Drug Name _____

Prescribed for: (Flu, pain, etc) _____

Dosage _____ Schedule _____ Pharmacy_____

Did medicine cure the problem? Y N Would I use it again? Y N

List any side effects _____

This medicine was prescribed during the doctor visit on page_____

Date _____

Drug Name _____

Prescribed for: (Flu, pain, etc) _____

Dosage _____ Schedule _____ Pharmacy _____

Did medicine cure the problem? Y N   Would I use it again? Y N

List any side effects _____

This medicine was prescribed during the doctor visit on page _____

Date _____

Drug Name _____

Prescribed for: (Flu, pain, etc) _____

Dosage _____ Schedule _____ Pharmacy _____

Did medicine cure the problem? Y N   Would I use it again? Y N

List any side effects _____

This medicine was prescribed during the doctor visit on page _____

Date _____

Drug Name _____

Prescribed for: (Flu, pain, etc) _____

Dosage _____ Schedule _____ Pharmacy _____

Did medicine cure the problem? Y N   Would I use it again? Y N

List any side effects _____

This medicine was prescribed during the doctor visit on page _____

Date _____

Drug Name _____

Prescribed for: (Flu, pain, etc) _____

Dosage _____ Schedule _____ Pharmacy _____

Did medicine cure the problem? Y N   Would I use it again? Y N

List any side effects _____

This medicine was prescribed during the doctor visit on page _____

Date

Drug Name _____

Prescribed for: (Flu, pain, etc) _____

Dosage _____ Schedule _____ Pharmacy_____

Did medicine cure the problem? Y N   Would I use it again? Y N

List any side effects _____

This medicine was prescribed during the doctor visit on page____

Date

Drug Name _____

Prescribed for: (Flu, pain, etc) _____

Dosage _____ Schedule _____ Pharmacy_____

Did medicine cure the problem? Y N   Would I use it again? Y N

List any side effects _____

This medicine was prescribed during the doctor visit on page____

Date

Drug Name _____

Prescribed for: (Flu, pain, etc) _____

Dosage _____ Schedule _____ Pharmacy_____

Did medicine cure the problem? Y N   Would I use it again? Y N

List any side effects _____

This medicine was prescribed during the doctor visit on page____

Date

Drug Name _____

Prescribed for: (Flu, pain, etc) _____

Dosage _____ Schedule _____ Pharmacy_____

Did medicine cure the problem? Y N   Would I use it again? Y N

List any side effects _____

This medicine was prescribed during the doctor visit on page____

J

Date _____

Drug Name _____

Prescribed for: (Flu, pain, etc) _____

Dosage _____ Schedule _____ Pharmacy _____

Did medicine cure the problem? Y N Would I use it again? Y N

List any side effects _____

This medicine was prescribed during the doctor visit on page _____

Date _____

Drug Name _____

Prescribed for: (Flu, pain, etc) _____

Dosage _____ Schedule _____ Pharmacy _____

Did medicine cure the problem? Y N Would I use it again? Y N

List any side effects _____

This medicine was prescribed during the doctor visit on page _____

Date _____

Drug Name _____

Prescribed for: (Flu, pain, etc) _____

Dosage _____ Schedule _____ Pharmacy _____

Did medicine cure the problem? Y N Would I use it again? Y N

List any side effects _____

This medicine was prescribed during the doctor visit on page _____

Date _____

Drug Name _____

Prescribed for: (Flu, pain, etc) _____

Dosage _____ Schedule _____ Pharmacy _____

Did medicine cure the problem? Y N Would I use it again? Y N

List any side effects _____

This medicine was prescribed during the doctor visit on page _____

Date _____ **J**

Drug Name _____

Prescribed for: (Flu, pain, etc) _____

Dosage _____ Schedule _____ Pharmacy_____

Did medicine cure the problem? Y N Would I use it again? Y N

List any side effects _____

This medicine was prescribed during the doctor visit on page_____

Date _____

Drug Name _____

Prescribed for: (Flu, pain, etc) _____

Dosage _____ Schedule _____ Pharmacy_____

Did medicine cure the problem? Y N Would I use it again? Y N

List any side effects _____

This medicine was prescribed during the doctor visit on page_____

Date _____

Drug Name _____

Prescribed for: (Flu, pain, etc) _____

Dosage _____ Schedule _____ Pharmacy_____

Did medicine cure the problem? Y N Would I use it again? Y N

List any side effects _____

This medicine was prescribed during the doctor visit on page_____

Date _____

Drug Name _____

Prescribed for: (Flu, pain, etc) _____

Dosage _____ Schedule _____ Pharmacy_____

Did medicine cure the problem? Y N Would I use it again? Y N

List any side effects _____

This medicine was prescribed during the doctor visit on page_____

K

Date _____

Drug Name _____

Prescribed for: (Flu, pain, etc) _____

Dosage _____ Schedule _____ Pharmacy _____

Did medicine cure the problem? Y N   Would I use it again? Y N

List any side effects _____

This medicine was prescribed during the doctor visit on page _____

Date _____

Drug Name _____

Prescribed for: (Flu, pain, etc) _____

Dosage _____ Schedule _____ Pharmacy _____

Did medicine cure the problem? Y N   Would I use it again? Y N

List any side effects _____

This medicine was prescribed during the doctor visit on page _____

Date _____

Drug Name _____

Prescribed for: (Flu, pain, etc) _____

Dosage _____ Schedule _____ Pharmacy _____

Did medicine cure the problem? Y N   Would I use it again? Y N

List any side effects _____

This medicine was prescribed during the doctor visit on page _____

Date _____

Drug Name _____

Prescribed for: (Flu, pain, etc) _____

Dosage _____ Schedule _____ Pharmacy _____

Did medicine cure the problem? Y N   Would I use it again? Y N

List any side effects _____

This medicine was prescribed during the doctor visit on page _____

K

Date _____

Drug Name _____

Prescribed for: (Flu, pain, etc) _____

Dosage _____ Schedule _____ Pharmacy _____

Did medicine cure the problem? Y N   Would I use it again? Y N

List any side effects _____

This medicine was prescribed during the doctor visit on page _____

Date _____

Drug Name _____

Prescribed for: (Flu, pain, etc) _____

Dosage _____ Schedule _____ Pharmacy _____

Did medicine cure the problem? Y N   Would I use it again? Y N

List any side effects _____

This medicine was prescribed during the doctor visit on page _____

Date _____

Drug Name _____

Prescribed for: (Flu, pain, etc) _____

Dosage _____ Schedule _____ Pharmacy _____

Did medicine cure the problem? Y N   Would I use it again? Y N

List any side effects _____

This medicine was prescribed during the doctor visit on page _____

Date _____

Drug Name _____

Prescribed for: (Flu, pain, etc) _____

Dosage _____ Schedule _____ Pharmacy _____

Did medicine cure the problem? Y N   Would I use it again? Y N

List any side effects _____

This medicine was prescribed during the doctor visit on page _____

L

Date _____

Drug Name _____

Prescribed for: (Flu, pain, etc) _____

Dosage _____ Schedule _____ Pharmacy _____

Did medicine cure the problem? Y N Would I use it again? Y N

List any side effects _____

This medicine was prescribed during the doctor visit on page _____

Date _____

Drug Name _____

Prescribed for: (Flu, pain, etc) _____

Dosage _____ Schedule _____ Pharmacy _____

Did medicine cure the problem? Y N Would I use it again? Y N

List any side effects _____

This medicine was prescribed during the doctor visit on page _____

Date _____

Drug Name _____

Prescribed for: (Flu, pain, etc) _____

Dosage _____ Schedule _____ Pharmacy _____

Did medicine cure the problem? Y N Would I use it again? Y N

List any side effects _____

This medicine was prescribed during the doctor visit on page _____

Date _____

Drug Name _____

Prescribed for: (Flu, pain, etc) _____

Dosage _____ Schedule _____ Pharmacy _____

Did medicine cure the problem? Y N Would I use it again? Y N

List any side effects _____

This medicine was prescribed during the doctor visit on page _____

L

Date _____

Drug Name _____

Prescribed for: (Flu, pain, etc) _____

Dosage _____ Schedule _____ Pharmacy _____

Did medicine cure the problem? Y N   Would I use it again? Y N

List any side effects _____

This medicine was prescribed during the doctor visit on page _____

Date _____

Drug Name _____

Prescribed for: (Flu, pain, etc) _____

Dosage _____ Schedule _____ Pharmacy _____

Did medicine cure the problem? Y N   Would I use it again? Y N

List any side effects _____

This medicine was prescribed during the doctor visit on page _____

Date _____

Drug Name _____

Prescribed for: (Flu, pain, etc) _____

Dosage _____ Schedule _____ Pharmacy _____

Did medicine cure the problem? Y N   Would I use it again? Y N

List any side effects _____

This medicine was prescribed during the doctor visit on page _____

Date _____

Drug Name _____

Prescribed for: (Flu, pain, etc) _____

Dosage _____ Schedule _____ Pharmacy _____

Did medicine cure the problem? Y N   Would I use it again? Y N

List any side effects _____

This medicine was prescribed during the doctor visit on page _____

M

Date

Drug Name _____

Prescribed for: (Flu, pain, etc) _____

Dosage _____ Schedule _____ Pharmacy_____

Did medicine cure the problem? Y N   Would I use it again? Y N

List any side effects _____

This medicine was prescribed during the doctor visit on page_____

Date

Drug Name _____

Prescribed for: (Flu, pain, etc) _____

Dosage _____ Schedule _____ Pharmacy_____

Did medicine cure the problem? Y N   Would I use it again? Y N

List any side effects _____

This medicine was prescribed during the doctor visit on page_____

Date

Drug Name _____

Prescribed for: (Flu, pain, etc) _____

Dosage _____ Schedule _____ Pharmacy_____

Did medicine cure the problem? Y N   Would I use it again? Y N

List any side effects _____

This medicine was prescribed during the doctor visit on page_____

Date

Drug Name _____

Prescribed for: (Flu, pain, etc) _____

Dosage _____ Schedule _____ Pharmacy_____

Did medicine cure the problem? Y N   Would I use it again? Y N

List any side effects _____

This medicine was prescribed during the doctor visit on page_____

Date _____ **M**

Drug Name _____

Prescribed for: (Flu, pain, etc) _____

Dosage _____ Schedule _____ Pharmacy _____

Did medicine cure the problem? Y N Would I use it again? Y N

List any side effects _____

This medicine was prescribed during the doctor visit on page _____

Date _____

Drug Name _____

Prescribed for: (Flu, pain, etc) _____

Dosage _____ Schedule _____ Pharmacy _____

Did medicine cure the problem? Y N Would I use it again? Y N

List any side effects _____

This medicine was prescribed during the doctor visit on page _____

Date _____

Drug Name _____

Prescribed for: (Flu, pain, etc) _____

Dosage _____ Schedule _____ Pharmacy _____

Did medicine cure the problem? Y N Would I use it again? Y N

List any side effects _____

This medicine was prescribed during the doctor visit on page _____

Date _____

Drug Name _____

Prescribed for: (Flu, pain, etc) _____

Dosage _____ Schedule _____ Pharmacy _____

Did medicine cure the problem? Y N Would I use it again? Y N

List any side effects _____

This medicine was prescribed during the doctor visit on page _____

N

Date _____

Drug Name _____

Prescribed for: (Flu, pain, etc) _____

Dosage _____ Schedule _____ Pharmacy_____

Did medicine cure the problem? Y N   Would I use it again? Y N

List any side effects _____

This medicine was prescribed during the doctor visit on page____

Date _____

Drug Name _____

Prescribed for: (Flu, pain, etc) _____

Dosage _____ Schedule _____ Pharmacy_____

Did medicine cure the problem? Y N   Would I use it again? Y N

List any side effects _____

This medicine was prescribed during the doctor visit on page____

Date _____

Drug Name _____

Prescribed for: (Flu, pain, etc) _____

Dosage _____ Schedule _____ Pharmacy_____

Did medicine cure the problem? Y N   Would I use it again? Y N

List any side effects _____

This medicine was prescribed during the doctor visit on page____

Date _____

Drug Name _____

Prescribed for: (Flu, pain, etc) _____

Dosage _____ Schedule _____ Pharmacy_____

Did medicine cure the problem? Y N   Would I use it again? Y N

List any side effects _____

This medicine was prescribed during the doctor visit on page____

Date _____

Drug Name _____

Prescribed for: (Flu, pain, etc) _____

Dosage _____ Schedule _____ Pharmacy_____

Did medicine cure the problem? Y N Would I use it again? Y N

List any side effects _____

This medicine was prescribed during the doctor visit on page_____

Date _____

Drug Name _____

Prescribed for: (Flu, pain, etc) _____

Dosage _____ Schedule _____ Pharmacy_____

Did medicine cure the problem? Y N Would I use it again? Y N

List any side effects _____

This medicine was prescribed during the doctor visit on page_____

Date _____

Drug Name _____

Prescribed for: (Flu, pain, etc) _____

Dosage _____ Schedule _____ Pharmacy_____

Did medicine cure the problem? Y N Would I use it again? Y N

List any side effects _____

This medicine was prescribed during the doctor visit on page_____

Date _____

Drug Name _____

Prescribed for: (Flu, pain, etc) _____

Dosage _____ Schedule _____ Pharmacy_____

Did medicine cure the problem? Y N Would I use it again? Y N

List any side effects _____

This medicine was prescribed during the doctor visit on page_____

O

Date _____

Drug Name _____

Prescribed for: (Flu, pain, etc) _____

Dosage _____ Schedule _____ Pharmacy _____

Did medicine cure the problem? Y N Would I use it again? Y N

List any side effects _____

This medicine was prescribed during the doctor visit on page _____

Date _____

Drug Name _____

Prescribed for: (Flu, pain, etc) _____

Dosage _____ Schedule _____ Pharmacy _____

Did medicine cure the problem? Y N Would I use it again? Y N

List any side effects _____

This medicine was prescribed during the doctor visit on page _____

Date _____

Drug Name _____

Prescribed for: (Flu, pain, etc) _____

Dosage _____ Schedule _____ Pharmacy _____

Did medicine cure the problem? Y N Would I use it again? Y N

List any side effects _____

This medicine was prescribed during the doctor visit on page _____

Date _____

Drug Name _____

Prescribed for: (Flu, pain, etc) _____

Dosage _____ Schedule _____ Pharmacy _____

Did medicine cure the problem? Y N Would I use it again? Y N

List any side effects _____

This medicine was prescribed during the doctor visit on page _____

Date _____ **O**

Drug Name _____

Prescribed for: (Flu, pain, etc) _____

Dosage _____ Schedule _____ Pharmacy_____

Did medicine cure the problem? Y N   Would I use it again? Y N

List any side effects _____

This medicine was prescribed during the doctor visit on page_____

Date _____

Drug Name _____

Prescribed for: (Flu, pain, etc) _____

Dosage _____ Schedule _____ Pharmacy_____

Did medicine cure the problem? Y N   Would I use it again? Y N

List any side effects _____

This medicine was prescribed during the doctor visit on page_____

Date _____

Drug Name _____

Prescribed for: (Flu, pain, etc) _____

Dosage _____ Schedule _____ Pharmacy_____

Did medicine cure the problem? Y N   Would I use it again? Y N

List any side effects _____

This medicine was prescribed during the doctor visit on page_____

Date _____

Drug Name _____

Prescribed for: (Flu, pain, etc) _____

Dosage _____ Schedule _____ Pharmacy_____

Did medicine cure the problem? Y N   Would I use it again? Y N

List any side effects _____

This medicine was prescribed during the doctor visit on page_____

P

Date _____

Drug Name _____

Prescribed for: (Flu, pain, etc) _____

Dosage _____ Schedule _____ Pharmacy_____

Did medicine cure the problem? Y N Would I use it again? Y N

List any side effects _____

This medicine was prescribed during the doctor visit on page_____

Date _____

Drug Name _____

Prescribed for: (Flu, pain, etc) _____

Dosage _____ Schedule _____ Pharmacy_____

Did medicine cure the problem? Y N Would I use it again? Y N

List any side effects _____

This medicine was prescribed during the doctor visit on page_____

Date _____

Drug Name _____

Prescribed for: (Flu, pain, etc) _____

Dosage _____ Schedule _____ Pharmacy_____

Did medicine cure the problem? Y N Would I use it again? Y N

List any side effects _____

This medicine was prescribed during the doctor visit on page_____

Date _____

Drug Name _____

Prescribed for: (Flu, pain, etc) _____

Dosage _____ Schedule _____ Pharmacy_____

Did medicine cure the problem? Y N Would I use it again? Y N

List any side effects _____

This medicine was prescribed during the doctor visit on page_____

P

Date _____

Drug Name _____

Prescribed for: (Flu, pain, etc) _____

Dosage _____ Schedule _____ Pharmacy _____

Did medicine cure the problem? Y N Would I use it again? Y N

List any side effects _____

This medicine was prescribed during the doctor visit on page _____

Date _____

Drug Name _____

Prescribed for: (Flu, pain, etc) _____

Dosage _____ Schedule _____ Pharmacy _____

Did medicine cure the problem? Y N Would I use it again? Y N

List any side effects _____

This medicine was prescribed during the doctor visit on page _____

Date _____

Drug Name _____

Prescribed for: (Flu, pain, etc) _____

Dosage _____ Schedule _____ Pharmacy _____

Did medicine cure the problem? Y N Would I use it again? Y N

List any side effects _____

This medicine was prescribed during the doctor visit on page _____

Date _____

Drug Name _____

Prescribed for: (Flu, pain, etc) _____

Dosage _____ Schedule _____ Pharmacy _____

Did medicine cure the problem? Y N Would I use it again? Y N

List any side effects _____

This medicine was prescribed during the doctor visit on page _____

Q

Date _____

Drug Name _____

Prescribed for: (Flu, pain, etc) _____

Dosage _____ Schedule _____ Pharmacy _____

Did medicine cure the problem? Y N   Would I use it again? Y N

List any side effects _____

This medicine was prescribed during the doctor visit on page _____

Date _____

Drug Name _____

Prescribed for: (Flu, pain, etc) _____

Dosage _____ Schedule _____ Pharmacy _____

Did medicine cure the problem? Y N   Would I use it again? Y N

List any side effects _____

This medicine was prescribed during the doctor visit on page _____

Date _____

Drug Name _____

Prescribed for: (Flu, pain, etc) _____

Dosage _____ Schedule _____ Pharmacy _____

Did medicine cure the problem? Y N   Would I use it again? Y N

List any side effects _____

This medicine was prescribed during the doctor visit on page _____

Date _____

Drug Name _____

Prescribed for: (Flu, pain, etc) _____

Dosage _____ Schedule _____ Pharmacy _____

Did medicine cure the problem? Y N   Would I use it again? Y N

List any side effects _____

This medicine was prescribed during the doctor visit on page _____

Date _____

Drug Name _____

Prescribed for: (Flu, pain, etc) _____

Dosage _____ Schedule _____ Pharmacy _____

Did medicine cure the problem? Y N   Would I use it again? Y N

List any side effects _____

This medicine was prescribed during the doctor visit on page_____

Date _____

Drug Name _____

Prescribed for: (Flu, pain, etc) _____

Dosage _____ Schedule _____ Pharmacy _____

Did medicine cure the problem? Y N   Would I use it again? Y N

List any side effects _____

This medicine was prescribed during the doctor visit on page_____

Date _____

Drug Name _____

Prescribed for: (Flu, pain, etc) _____

Dosage _____ Schedule _____ Pharmacy _____

Did medicine cure the problem? Y N   Would I use it again? Y N

List any side effects _____

This medicine was prescribed during the doctor visit on page_____

Date _____

Drug Name _____

Prescribed for: (Flu, pain, etc) _____

Dosage _____ Schedule _____ Pharmacy _____

Did medicine cure the problem? Y N   Would I use it again? Y N

List any side effects _____

This medicine was prescribed during the doctor visit on page_____

R
Date _____

Drug Name _____
Prescribed for: (Flu, pain, etc) _____
Dosage _____ Schedule _____ Pharmacy _____
Did medicine cure the problem? Y N   Would I use it again? Y N
List any side effects _____

This medicine was prescribed during the doctor visit on page _____

Date _____

Drug Name _____
Prescribed for: (Flu, pain, etc) _____
Dosage _____ Schedule _____ Pharmacy _____
Did medicine cure the problem? Y N   Would I use it again? Y N
List any side effects _____

This medicine was prescribed during the doctor visit on page _____

Date _____

Drug Name _____
Prescribed for: (Flu, pain, etc) _____
Dosage _____ Schedule _____ Pharmacy _____
Did medicine cure the problem? Y N   Would I use it again? Y N
List any side effects _____

This medicine was prescribed during the doctor visit on page _____

Date _____

Drug Name _____
Prescribed for: (Flu, pain, etc) _____
Dosage _____ Schedule _____ Pharmacy _____
Did medicine cure the problem? Y N   Would I use it again? Y N
List any side effects _____

This medicine was prescribed during the doctor visit on page _____

R

Date _____

Drug Name _____

Prescribed for: (Flu, pain, etc) _____

Dosage _____ Schedule _____ Pharmacy _____

Did medicine cure the problem? Y N   Would I use it again? Y N

List any side effects _____

This medicine was prescribed during the doctor visit on page _____

Date _____

Drug Name _____

Prescribed for: (Flu, pain, etc) _____

Dosage _____ Schedule _____ Pharmacy _____

Did medicine cure the problem? Y N   Would I use it again? Y N

List any side effects _____

This medicine was prescribed during the doctor visit on page _____

Date _____

Drug Name _____

Prescribed for: (Flu, pain, etc) _____

Dosage _____ Schedule _____ Pharmacy _____

Did medicine cure the problem? Y N   Would I use it again? Y N

List any side effects _____

This medicine was prescribed during the doctor visit on page _____

Date _____

Drug Name _____

Prescribed for: (Flu, pain, etc) _____

Dosage _____ Schedule _____ Pharmacy _____

Did medicine cure the problem? Y N   Would I use it again? Y N

List any side effects _____

This medicine was prescribed during the doctor visit on page _____

S

Drug Name _____

Prescribed for: (Flu, pain, etc) _____

Dosage _____ Schedule _____ Pharmacy_____

Did medicine cure the problem? Y N Would I use it again? Y N

List any side effects _____

This medicine was prescribed during the doctor visit on page_____

Date

Drug Name _____

Prescribed for: (Flu, pain, etc) _____

Dosage _____ Schedule _____ Pharmacy_____

Did medicine cure the problem? Y N Would I use it again? Y N

List any side effects _____

This medicine was prescribed during the doctor visit on page_____

Date

Drug Name _____

Prescribed for: (Flu, pain, etc) _____

Dosage _____ Schedule _____ Pharmacy_____

Did medicine cure the problem? Y N Would I use it again? Y N

List any side effects _____

This medicine was prescribed during the doctor visit on page_____

Date

Drug Name _____

Prescribed for: (Flu, pain, etc) _____

Dosage _____ Schedule _____ Pharmacy_____

Did medicine cure the problem? Y N Would I use it again? Y N

List any side effects _____

This medicine was prescribed during the doctor visit on page_____

Drug Name _____

Prescribed for: (Flu, pain, etc) _____

Dosage _____ Schedule _____ Pharmacy_____

Did medicine cure the problem? Y N   Would I use it again? Y N

List any side effects _____

This medicine was prescribed during the doctor visit on page____

Date

Drug Name _____

Prescribed for: (Flu, pain, etc) _____

Dosage _____ Schedule _____ Pharmacy_____

Did medicine cure the problem? Y N   Would I use it again? Y N

List any side effects _____

This medicine was prescribed during the doctor visit on page____

Date

Drug Name _____

Prescribed for: (Flu, pain, etc) _____

Dosage _____ Schedule _____ Pharmacy_____

Did medicine cure the problem? Y N   Would I use it again? Y N

List any side effects _____

This medicine was prescribed during the doctor visit on page____

Date

Drug Name _____

Prescribed for: (Flu, pain, etc) _____

Dosage _____ Schedule _____ Pharmacy_____

Did medicine cure the problem? Y N   Would I use it again? Y N

List any side effects _____

This medicine was prescribed during the doctor visit on page____

T

Date _____

Drug Name _____

Prescribed for: (Flu, pain, etc) _____

Dosage _____ Schedule _____ Pharmacy_____

Did medicine cure the problem? Y N   Would I use it again? Y N

List any side effects _____

This medicine was prescribed during the doctor visit on page_____

Date _____

Drug Name _____

Prescribed for: (Flu, pain, etc) _____

Dosage _____ Schedule _____ Pharmacy_____

Did medicine cure the problem? Y N   Would I use it again? Y N

List any side effects _____

This medicine was prescribed during the doctor visit on page_____

Date _____

Drug Name _____

Prescribed for: (Flu, pain, etc) _____

Dosage _____ Schedule _____ Pharmacy_____

Did medicine cure the problem? Y N   Would I use it again? Y N

List any side effects _____

This medicine was prescribed during the doctor visit on page_____

Date _____

Drug Name _____

Prescribed for: (Flu, pain, etc) _____

Dosage _____ Schedule _____ Pharmacy_____

Did medicine cure the problem? Y N   Would I use it again? Y N

List any side effects _____

This medicine was prescribed during the doctor visit on page_____

Date _____

Drug Name _____
Prescribed for: (Flu, pain, etc) _____
Dosage _____ Schedule _____ Pharmacy_____
Did medicine cure the problem? Y N   Would I use it again? Y N
List any side effects _____

This medicine was prescribed during the doctor visit on page_____

Date _____

Drug Name _____
Prescribed for: (Flu, pain, etc) _____
Dosage _____ Schedule _____ Pharmacy_____
Did medicine cure the problem? Y N   Would I use it again? Y N
List any side effects _____

This medicine was prescribed during the doctor visit on page_____

Date _____

Drug Name _____
Prescribed for: (Flu, pain, etc) _____
Dosage _____ Schedule _____ Pharmacy_____
Did medicine cure the problem? Y N   Would I use it again? Y N
List any side effects _____

This medicine was prescribed during the doctor visit on page_____

Date _____

Drug Name _____
Prescribed for: (Flu, pain, etc) _____
Dosage _____ Schedule _____ Pharmacy_____
Did medicine cure the problem? Y N   Would I use it again? Y N
List any side effects _____

This medicine was prescribed during the doctor visit on page_____

U

Date _____

Drug Name _____

Prescribed for: (Flu, pain, etc) _____

Dosage _____ Schedule _____ Pharmacy _____

Did medicine cure the problem? Y N   Would I use it again? Y N

List any side effects _____

This medicine was prescribed during the doctor visit on page _____

Date _____

Drug Name _____

Prescribed for: (Flu, pain, etc) _____

Dosage _____ Schedule _____ Pharmacy _____

Did medicine cure the problem? Y N   Would I use it again? Y N

List any side effects _____

This medicine was prescribed during the doctor visit on page _____

Date _____

Drug Name _____

Prescribed for: (Flu, pain, etc) _____

Dosage _____ Schedule _____ Pharmacy _____

Did medicine cure the problem? Y N   Would I use it again? Y N

List any side effects _____

This medicine was prescribed during the doctor visit on page _____

Date _____

Drug Name _____

Prescribed for: (Flu, pain, etc) _____

Dosage _____ Schedule _____ Pharmacy _____

Did medicine cure the problem? Y N   Would I use it again? Y N

List any side effects _____

This medicine was prescribed during the doctor visit on page _____

U

Date _____

Drug Name _____

Prescribed for: (Flu, pain, etc) _____

Dosage _____ Schedule _____ Pharmacy_____

Did medicine cure the problem? Y N Would I use it again? Y N

List any side effects _____

This medicine was prescribed during the doctor visit on page_____

Date _____

Drug Name _____

Prescribed for: (Flu, pain, etc) _____

Dosage _____ Schedule _____ Pharmacy_____

Did medicine cure the problem? Y N Would I use it again? Y N

List any side effects _____

This medicine was prescribed during the doctor visit on page_____

Date _____

Drug Name _____

Prescribed for: (Flu, pain, etc) _____

Dosage _____ Schedule _____ Pharmacy_____

Did medicine cure the problem? Y N Would I use it again? Y N

List any side effects _____

This medicine was prescribed during the doctor visit on page_____

Date _____

Drug Name _____

Prescribed for: (Flu, pain, etc) _____

Dosage _____ Schedule _____ Pharmacy_____

Did medicine cure the problem? Y N Would I use it again? Y N

List any side effects _____

This medicine was prescribed during the doctor visit on page_____

V

Date _____

Drug Name _____

Prescribed for: (Flu, pain, etc) _____

Dosage _____ Schedule _____ Pharmacy _____

Did medicine cure the problem? Y N   Would I use it again? Y N

List any side effects _____

This medicine was prescribed during the doctor visit on page _____

Date _____

Drug Name _____

Prescribed for: (Flu, pain, etc) _____

Dosage _____ Schedule _____ Pharmacy _____

Did medicine cure the problem? Y N   Would I use it again? Y N

List any side effects _____

This medicine was prescribed during the doctor visit on page _____

Date _____

Drug Name _____

Prescribed for: (Flu, pain, etc) _____

Dosage _____ Schedule _____ Pharmacy _____

Did medicine cure the problem? Y N   Would I use it again? Y N

List any side effects _____

This medicine was prescribed during the doctor visit on page _____

Date _____

Drug Name _____

Prescribed for: (Flu, pain, etc) _____

Dosage _____ Schedule _____ Pharmacy _____

Did medicine cure the problem? Y N   Would I use it again? Y N

List any side effects _____

This medicine was prescribed during the doctor visit on page _____

V

Date _____

Drug Name _____
Prescribed for: (Flu, pain, etc) _____
Dosage _____ Schedule _____ Pharmacy _____
Did medicine cure the problem? Y N   Would I use it again? Y N
List any side effects _____

This medicine was prescribed during the doctor visit on page _____

Date _____

Drug Name _____
Prescribed for: (Flu, pain, etc) _____
Dosage _____ Schedule _____ Pharmacy _____
Did medicine cure the problem? Y N   Would I use it again? Y N
List any side effects _____

This medicine was prescribed during the doctor visit on page _____

Date _____

Drug Name _____
Prescribed for: (Flu, pain, etc) _____
Dosage _____ Schedule _____ Pharmacy _____
Did medicine cure the problem? Y N   Would I use it again? Y N
List any side effects _____

This medicine was prescribed during the doctor visit on page _____

Date _____

Drug Name _____
Prescribed for: (Flu, pain, etc) _____
Dosage _____ Schedule _____ Pharmacy _____
Did medicine cure the problem? Y N   Would I use it again? Y N
List any side effects _____

This medicine was prescribed during the doctor visit on page _____

W

Date

Drug Name _____

Prescribed for: (Flu, pain, etc) _____

Dosage _____ Schedule _____ Pharmacy _____

Did medicine cure the problem? Y N   Would I use it again? Y N

List any side effects _____

This medicine was prescribed during the doctor visit on page _____

Date

Drug Name _____

Prescribed for: (Flu, pain, etc) _____

Dosage _____ Schedule _____ Pharmacy _____

Did medicine cure the problem? Y N   Would I use it again? Y N

List any side effects _____

This medicine was prescribed during the doctor visit on page _____

Date

Drug Name _____

Prescribed for: (Flu, pain, etc) _____

Dosage _____ Schedule _____ Pharmacy _____

Did medicine cure the problem? Y N   Would I use it again? Y N

List any side effects _____

This medicine was prescribed during the doctor visit on page _____

Date

Drug Name _____

Prescribed for: (Flu, pain, etc) _____

Dosage _____ Schedule _____ Pharmacy _____

Did medicine cure the problem? Y N   Would I use it again? Y N

List any side effects _____

This medicine was prescribed during the doctor visit on page _____

W

Date _____

Drug Name _____

Prescribed for: (Flu, pain, etc) _____

Dosage _____ Schedule _____ Pharmacy _____

Did medicine cure the problem? Y N Would I use it again? Y N

List any side effects _____

This medicine was prescribed during the doctor visit on page _____

Date _____

Drug Name _____

Prescribed for: (Flu, pain, etc) _____

Dosage _____ Schedule _____ Pharmacy _____

Did medicine cure the problem? Y N Would I use it again? Y N

List any side effects _____

This medicine was prescribed during the doctor visit on page _____

Date _____

Drug Name _____

Prescribed for: (Flu, pain, etc) _____

Dosage _____ Schedule _____ Pharmacy _____

Did medicine cure the problem? Y N Would I use it again? Y N

List any side effects _____

This medicine was prescribed during the doctor visit on page _____

Date _____

Drug Name _____

Prescribed for: (Flu, pain, etc) _____

Dosage _____ Schedule _____ Pharmacy _____

Did medicine cure the problem? Y N Would I use it again? Y N

List any side effects _____

This medicine was prescribed during the doctor visit on page _____

X

Date _____

Drug Name _____

Prescribed for: (Flu, pain, etc) _____

Dosage _____Schedule _____ Pharmacy_____

Did medicine cure the problem? Y N Would I use it again? Y N

List any side effects _____

This medicine was prescribed during the doctor visit on page_____

Date _____

Drug Name _____

Prescribed for: (Flu, pain, etc) _____

Dosage _____Schedule _____ Pharmacy_____

Did medicine cure the problem? Y N Would I use it again? Y N

List any side effects _____

This medicine was prescribed during the doctor visit on page_____

Date _____

Drug Name _____

Prescribed for: (Flu, pain, etc) _____

Dosage _____Schedule _____ Pharmacy_____

Did medicine cure the problem? Y N Would I use it again? Y N

List any side effects _____

This medicine was prescribed during the doctor visit on page_____

Date _____

Drug Name _____

Prescribed for: (Flu, pain, etc) _____

Dosage _____Schedule _____ Pharmacy_____

Did medicine cure the problem? Y N Would I use it again? Y N

List any side effects _____

This medicine was prescribed during the doctor visit on page_____

X

Date _____

Drug Name _____

Prescribed for: (Flu, pain, etc) _____

Dosage _____ Schedule _____ Pharmacy_____

Did medicine cure the problem? Y N   Would I use it again? Y N

List any side effects _____

This medicine was prescribed during the doctor visit on page_____

Date _____

Drug Name _____

Prescribed for: (Flu, pain, etc) _____

Dosage _____ Schedule _____ Pharmacy_____

Did medicine cure the problem? Y N   Would I use it again? Y N

List any side effects _____

This medicine was prescribed during the doctor visit on page_____

Date _____

Drug Name _____

Prescribed for: (Flu, pain, etc) _____

Dosage _____ Schedule _____ Pharmacy_____

Did medicine cure the problem? Y N   Would I use it again? Y N

List any side effects _____

This medicine was prescribed during the doctor visit on page_____

Date _____

Drug Name _____

Prescribed for: (Flu, pain, etc) _____

Dosage _____ Schedule _____ Pharmacy_____

Did medicine cure the problem? Y N   Would I use it again? Y N

List any side effects _____

This medicine was prescribed during the doctor visit on page_____

Y

Date _____

Drug Name _____
Prescribed for: (Flu, pain, etc) _____
Dosage _____ Schedule _____ Pharmacy _____
Did medicine cure the problem? Y N   Would I use it again? Y N
List any side effects _____

This medicine was prescribed during the doctor visit on page _____

Date _____

Drug Name _____
Prescribed for: (Flu, pain, etc) _____
Dosage _____ Schedule _____ Pharmacy _____
Did medicine cure the problem? Y N   Would I use it again? Y N
List any side effects _____

This medicine was prescribed during the doctor visit on page _____

Date _____

Drug Name _____
Prescribed for: (Flu, pain, etc) _____
Dosage _____ Schedule _____ Pharmacy _____
Did medicine cure the problem? Y N   Would I use it again? Y N
List any side effects _____

This medicine was prescribed during the doctor visit on page _____

Date _____

Drug Name _____
Prescribed for: (Flu, pain, etc) _____
Dosage _____ Schedule _____ Pharmacy _____
Did medicine cure the problem? Y N   Would I use it again? Y N
List any side effects _____

This medicine was prescribed during the doctor visit on page _____

Y

Date _____

Drug Name _____
Prescribed for: (Flu, pain, etc) _____
Dosage _____ Schedule _____ Pharmacy _____
Did medicine cure the problem? Y N   Would I use it again? Y N
List any side effects _____

This medicine was prescribed during the doctor visit on page _____

Date _____

Drug Name _____
Prescribed for: (Flu, pain, etc) _____
Dosage _____ Schedule _____ Pharmacy _____
Did medicine cure the problem? Y N   Would I use it again? Y N
List any side effects _____

This medicine was prescribed during the doctor visit on page _____

Date _____

Drug Name _____
Prescribed for: (Flu, pain, etc) _____
Dosage _____ Schedule _____ Pharmacy _____
Did medicine cure the problem? Y N   Would I use it again? Y N
List any side effects _____

This medicine was prescribed during the doctor visit on page _____

Date _____

Drug Name _____
Prescribed for: (Flu, pain, etc) _____
Dosage _____ Schedule _____ Pharmacy _____
Did medicine cure the problem? Y N   Would I use it again? Y N
List any side effects _____

This medicine was prescribed during the doctor visit on page _____

Z

Date _____

Drug Name _____

Prescribed for: (Flu, pain, etc) _____

Dosage _____ Schedule _____ Pharmacy _____

Did medicine cure the problem? Y N Would I use it again? Y N

List any side effects _____

This medicine was prescribed during the doctor visit on page _____

Date _____

Drug Name _____

Prescribed for: (Flu, pain, etc) _____

Dosage _____ Schedule _____ Pharmacy _____

Did medicine cure the problem? Y N Would I use it again? Y N

List any side effects _____

This medicine was prescribed during the doctor visit on page _____

Date _____

Drug Name _____

Prescribed for: (Flu, pain, etc) _____

Dosage _____ Schedule _____ Pharmacy _____

Did medicine cure the problem? Y N Would I use it again? Y N

List any side effects _____

This medicine was prescribed during the doctor visit on page _____

Date _____

Drug Name _____

Prescribed for: (Flu, pain, etc) _____

Dosage _____ Schedule _____ Pharmacy _____

Did medicine cure the problem? Y N Would I use it again? Y N

List any side effects _____

This medicine was prescribed during the doctor visit on page _____

Z

Date _____

Drug Name _____

Prescribed for: (Flu, pain, etc) _____

Dosage _____ Schedule _____ Pharmacy _____

Did medicine cure the problem? Y N   Would I use it again? Y N

List any side effects _____

This medicine was prescribed during the doctor visit on page _____

Date _____

Drug Name _____

Prescribed for: (Flu, pain, etc) _____

Dosage _____ Schedule _____ Pharmacy _____

Did medicine cure the problem? Y N   Would I use it again? Y N

List any side effects _____

This medicine was prescribed during the doctor visit on page _____

Date _____

Drug Name _____

Prescribed for: (Flu, pain, etc) _____

Dosage _____ Schedule _____ Pharmacy _____

Did medicine cure the problem? Y N   Would I use it again? Y N

List any side effects _____

This medicine was prescribed during the doctor visit on page _____

Date _____

Drug Name _____

Prescribed for: (Flu, pain, etc) _____

Dosage _____ Schedule _____ Pharmacy _____

Did medicine cure the problem? Y N   Would I use it again? Y N

List any side effects _____

This medicine was prescribed during the doctor visit on page _____

SCANS

Use this section to keep up with MRI's, CT's, Ultrasounds, Mammograms, etc.

The first MRI scan performed on the human body was conducted in 1971. Today, more than 37 million MRIs are done in the United States each year.

Did you know that x-rays were discovered by accident?

William Roentgen was a German physicist who was studying the pathways of electricity in 1895. His wife put her hand on the photographic plate in the pathway of then-unknown x-rays. The first x-ray of her hand was achieved.

Upon seeing the image, his wife stated that 'she had seen her death!'

Roentgen won a Nobel Prize in Physics in 1901. He didn't patent his discoveries. He wanted all of mankind to benefit from them. Fictionistic.com and Wikipedia.com

Type of scan _____ Date_____

Doctor_____ Ph.# _____

Address where scan performed_____

Body area scanned_____

Reason for scan_____

Medication used during scan (IV, sedative etc.) _____

Adverse reaction during scan _____

Diagnosis from scan _____

Scan ordered during Doctor visit listed on page _____

Type of scan _____ Date_____

Doctor_____ Ph.# _____

Address where scan performed_____

Body area scanned_____

Reason for scan_____

Medication used during scan (IV, sedative etc.) _____

Adverse reaction during scan _____

Diagnosis from scan _____

Scan ordered during Doctor visit listed on page _____

Type of scan _____ Date_____

Doctor_____ Ph.# _____

Address where scan performed_____

Body area scanned_____

Reason for scan_____

Medication used during scan (IV, sedative etc.) _____

Adverse reaction during scan _____

Diagnosis from scan _____

Scan ordered during Doctor visit listed on page _____

Type of scan _____ Date_____

Doctor_____ Ph.# _____

Address where scan performed_____

Body area scanned_____

Reason for scan_____

Medication used during scan (IV, sedative etc.) _____

Adverse reaction during scan _____

Diagnosis from scan _____

Scan ordered during Doctor visit listed on page _____

Type of scan _____ Date_____

Doctor_____ Ph.# _____

Address where scan performed_____

Body area scanned_____

Reason for scan_____

Medication used during scan (IV, sedative etc.) _____

Adverse reaction during scan _____

Diagnosis from scan _____

Scan ordered during Doctor visit listed on page _____

Type of scan _____ Date_____

Doctor_____ Ph.# _____

Address where scan performed_____

Body area scanned_____

Reason for scan_____

Medication used during scan (IV, sedative etc.) _____

Adverse reaction during scan _____

Diagnosis from scan _____

Scan ordered during Doctor visit listed on page _____

Type of scan _____ Date_____

Doctor_____ Ph.# _____

Address where scan performed_____

Body area scanned_____

Reason for scan_____

Medication used during scan (IV, sedative etc.) _____

Adverse reaction during scan _____

Diagnosis from scan _____

Scan ordered during Doctor visit listed on page _____

Type of scan _____ Date_____

Doctor_____ Ph.# _____

Address where scan performed_____

Body area scanned_____

Reason for scan_____

Medication used during scan (IV, sedative etc.) _____

Adverse reaction during scan _____

Diagnosis from scan _____

Scan ordered during Doctor visit listed on page _____

Type of scan _____ Date_____

Doctor_____ Ph.# _____

Address where scan performed_____

Body area scanned_____

Reason for scan_____

Medication used during scan (IV, sedative etc.) _____

Adverse reaction during scan _____

Diagnosis from scan _____

Scan ordered during Doctor visit listed on page _____

Type of scan _____Date_____

Doctor_____ Ph.# _____

Address where scan performed_____

Body area scanned_____

Reason for scan_____

Medication used during scan (IV, sedative etc.) _____

Adverse reaction during scan _____

Diagnosis from scan_____

Scan ordered during Doctor visit listed on page _____

Type of scan _____Date_____

Doctor_____ Ph.# _____

Address where scan performed_____

Body area scanned_____

Reason for scan_____

Medication used during scan (IV, sedative etc.) _____

Adverse reaction during scan _____

Diagnosis from scan_____

Scan ordered during Doctor visit listed on page _____

Type of scan _____Date_____

Doctor_____ Ph.# _____

Address where scan performed_____

Body area scanned_____

Reason for scan_____

Medication used during scan (IV, sedative etc.) _____

Adverse reaction during scan _____

Diagnosis from scan_____

Scan ordered during Doctor visit listed on page _____

Type of scan _____Date_____

Doctor_____ Ph.# _____

Address where scan performed _____

Body area scanned_____

Reason for scan_____

Medication used during scan (IV, sedative etc.) _____

Adverse reaction during scan _____

Diagnosis from scan _____

Scan ordered during Doctor visit listed on page _____

Type of scan _____Date_____

Doctor_____ Ph.# _____

Address where scan performed _____

Body area scanned_____

Reason for scan_____

Medication used during scan (IV, sedative etc.) _____

Adverse reaction during scan _____

Diagnosis from scan _____

Scan ordered during Doctor visit listed on page _____

Type of scan _____Date_____

Doctor_____ Ph.# _____

Address where scan performed _____

Body area scanned_____

Reason for scan_____

Medication used during scan (IV, sedative etc.) _____

Adverse reaction during scan _____

Diagnosis from scan _____

Scan ordered during Doctor visit listed on page _____

Type of scan _____Date_____

Doctor_____ Ph.# _____

Address where scan performed_____

Body area scanned_____

Reason for scan_____

Medication used during scan (IV, sedative etc.) _____

Adverse reaction during scan _____

Diagnosis from scan _____

Scan ordered during Doctor visit listed on page _____

Type of scan _____Date_____

Doctor_____ Ph.# _____

Address where scan performed_____

Body area scanned_____

Reason for scan_____

Medication used during scan (IV, sedative etc.) _____

Adverse reaction during scan _____

Diagnosis from scan _____

Scan ordered during Doctor visit listed on page _____

Type of scan _____Date_____

Doctor_____ Ph.# _____

Address where scan performed_____

Body area scanned_____

Reason for scan_____

Medication used during scan (IV, sedative etc.) _____

Adverse reaction during scan _____

Diagnosis from scan _____

Scan ordered during Doctor visit listed on page _____

Type of scan _____ Date_____

Doctor_____ Ph.# _____

Address where scan performed_____

Body area scanned_____

Reason for scan_____

Medication used during scan (IV, sedative etc.) _____

Adverse reaction during scan _____

Diagnosis from scan _____

Scan ordered during Doctor visit listed on page _____

Type of scan _____ Date_____

Doctor_____ Ph.# _____

Address where scan performed_____

Body area scanned_____

Reason for scan_____

Medication used during scan (IV, sedative etc.) _____

Adverse reaction during scan _____

Diagnosis from scan _____

Scan ordered during Doctor visit listed on page _____

Type of scan _____ Date_____

Doctor_____ Ph.# _____

Address where scan performed_____

Body area scanned_____

Reason for scan_____

Medication used during scan (IV, sedative etc.) _____

Adverse reaction during scan _____

Diagnosis from scan _____

Scan ordered during Doctor visit listed on page _____

Type of scan _____ Date_____

Doctor_____ Ph.# _____

Address where scan performed_____

Body area scanned_____

Reason for scan_____

Medication used during scan (IV, sedative etc.) _____

Adverse reaction during scan _____

Diagnosis from scan_____

Scan ordered during Doctor visit listed on page _____

Type of scan _____ Date_____

Doctor_____ Ph.# _____

Address where scan performed_____

Body area scanned_____

Reason for scan_____

Medication used during scan (IV, sedative etc.) _____

Adverse reaction during scan _____

Diagnosis from scan_____

Scan ordered during Doctor visit listed on page _____

Type of scan _____ Date_____

Doctor_____ Ph.# _____

Address where scan performed_____

Body area scanned_____

Reason for scan_____

Medication used during scan (IV, sedative etc.) _____

Adverse reaction during scan _____

Diagnosis from scan_____

Scan ordered during Doctor visit listed on page _____

Type of scan _____ Date_____

Doctor_____ Ph.# _____

Address where scan performed_____

Body area scanned_____

Reason for scan_____

Medication used during scan (IV, sedative etc.) _____

Adverse reaction during scan _____

Diagnosis from scan_____

Scan ordered during Doctor visit listed on page _____

Type of scan _____ Date_____

Doctor_____ Ph.# _____

Address where scan performed_____

Body area scanned_____

Reason for scan_____

Medication used during scan (IV, sedative etc.) _____

Adverse reaction during scan _____

Diagnosis from scan_____

Scan ordered during Doctor visit listed on page _____

Type of scan _____ Date_____

Doctor_____ Ph.# _____

Address where scan performed_____

Body area scanned_____

Reason for scan_____

Medication used during scan (IV, sedative etc.) _____

Adverse reaction during scan _____

Diagnosis from scan_____

Scan ordered during Doctor visit listed on page _____

Type of scan _____ Date_____

Doctor_____ Ph.# _____

Address where scan performed_____

Body area scanned_____

Reason for scan_____

Medication used during scan (IV, sedative etc.) _____

Adverse reaction during scan _____

Diagnosis from scan_____

Scan ordered during Doctor visit listed on page _____

Type of scan _____ Date_____

Doctor_____ Ph.# _____

Address where scan performed_____

Body area scanned_____

Reason for scan_____

Medication used during scan (IV, sedative etc.) _____

Adverse reaction during scan _____

Diagnosis from scan_____

Scan ordered during Doctor visit listed on page _____

Type of scan _____ Date_____

Doctor_____ Ph.# _____

Address where scan performed_____

Body area scanned_____

Reason for scan_____

Medication used during scan (IV, sedative etc.) _____

Adverse reaction during scan _____

Diagnosis from scan_____

Scan ordered during Doctor visit listed on page _____

Type of scan _____ Date_____

Doctor_____ Ph.# _____

Address where scan performed _____

Body area scanned_____

Reason for scan_____

Medication used during scan (IV, sedative etc.) _____

Adverse reaction during scan _____

Diagnosis from scan _____

Scan ordered during Doctor visit listed on page _____

Type of scan _____ Date_____

Doctor_____ Ph.# _____

Address where scan performed _____

Body area scanned_____

Reason for scan_____

Medication used during scan (IV, sedative etc.) _____

Adverse reaction during scan _____

Diagnosis from scan _____

Scan ordered during Doctor visit listed on page _____

Type of scan _____ Date_____

Doctor_____ Ph.# _____

Address where scan performed _____

Body area scanned_____

Reason for scan_____

Medication used during scan (IV, sedative etc.) _____

Adverse reaction during scan _____

Diagnosis from scan _____

Scan ordered during Doctor visit listed on page _____

Type of scan _____ Date_____

Doctor_____ Ph.# _____

Address where scan performed_____

Body area scanned_____

Reason for scan_____

Medication used during scan (IV, sedative etc.) _____

Adverse reaction during scan _____

Diagnosis from scan _____

Scan ordered during Doctor visit listed on page _____

Type of scan _____ Date_____

Doctor_____ Ph.# _____

Address where scan performed_____

Body area scanned_____

Reason for scan_____

Medication used during scan (IV, sedative etc.) _____

Adverse reaction during scan _____

Diagnosis from scan _____

Scan ordered during Doctor visit listed on page _____

Type of scan _____ Date_____

Doctor_____ Ph.# _____

Address where scan performed_____

Body area scanned_____

Reason for scan_____

Medication used during scan (IV, sedative etc.) _____

Adverse reaction during scan _____

Diagnosis from scan _____

Scan ordered during Doctor visit listed on page _____

Procedures

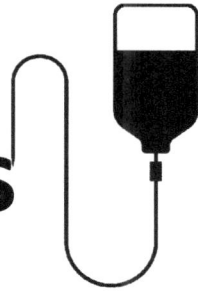

The total number of major procedures performed in the United States is estimated to be 51.4 million per year.

Most common?

Heart procedures including angiography and arteriography, cardiac catherizations, balloon angioplasty, insertion of coronary artery stent and coronary artery bypass graft.

The second most common is a cesarean section and hysterectomy.

And the third most common is in the orthopedic field including fracture, knee replacement and hip replacement

Procedure_____ Date_____
Doctor_____ Ph.# _____
Where was procedure performed?_____
Reason for procedure_____

Adverse reaction during or after procedure _____

Was procedure successful? Y N   Procedure needed again? Y N
Procedure ordered during Doctor visit listed on page _____

Procedure_____ Date_____
Doctor_____ Ph.# _____
Where was procedure performed?_____
Reason for procedure_____

Adverse reaction during or after procedure _____

Was procedure successful? Y N   Procedure needed again? Y N
Procedure ordered during Doctor visit listed on page _____

Procedure_____ Date_____
Doctor_____ Ph.# _____
Where was procedure performed?_____
Reason for procedure_____

Adverse reaction during or after procedure _____

Was procedure successful? Y N   Procedure needed again? Y N
Procedure ordered during Doctor visit listed on page _____

Procedure_____ Date_____

Doctor_____Ph.# _____

Where was procedure performed?_____

Reason for procedure_____

Adverse reaction during or after procedure _____

Was procedure successful? Y N Procedure needed again? Y N

Procedure ordered during Doctor visit listed on page _____

Procedure_____ Date_____

Doctor_____Ph.# _____

Where was procedure performed?_____

Reason for procedure_____

Adverse reaction during or after procedure _____

Was procedure successful? Y N Procedure needed again? Y N

Procedure ordered during Doctor visit listed on page _____

Procedure_____ Date_____

Doctor_____Ph.# _____

Where was procedure performed?_____

Reason for procedure_____

Adverse reaction during or after procedure _____

Was procedure successful? Y N Procedure needed again? Y N

Procedure ordered during Doctor visit listed on page _____

Procedure_____ Date_____

Doctor_____ Ph.# _____

Where was procedure performed?_____

Reason for procedure_____

Adverse reaction during or after procedure _____

Was procedure successful? Y N   Procedure needed again? Y   N

Procedure ordered during Doctor visit listed on page _____

Procedure_____ Date_____

Doctor_____ Ph.# _____

Where was procedure performed?_____

Reason for procedure_____

Adverse reaction during or after procedure _____

Was procedure successful? Y N   Procedure needed again? Y   N

Procedure ordered during Doctor visit listed on page _____

Procedure_____ Date_____

Doctor_____ Ph.# _____

Where was procedure performed?_____

Reason for procedure_____

Adverse reaction during or after procedure _____

Was procedure successful? Y N   Procedure needed again? Y   N

Procedure ordered during Doctor visit listed on page _____

Procedure_____ Date_____

Doctor_____Ph.# _____

Where was procedure performed?_____

Reason for procedure_____

Adverse reaction during or after procedure _____

Was procedure successful? Y N Procedure needed again? Y N

Procedure ordered during Doctor visit listed on page _____

Procedure_____ Date_____

Doctor_____Ph.# _____

Where was procedure performed?_____

Reason for procedure_____

Adverse reaction during or after procedure _____

Was procedure successful? Y N Procedure needed again? Y N

Procedure ordered during Doctor visit listed on page _____

Procedure_____ Date_____

Doctor_____Ph.# _____

Where was procedure performed?_____

Reason for procedure_____

Adverse reaction during or after procedure _____

Was procedure successful? Y N Procedure needed again? Y N

Procedure ordered during Doctor visit listed on page _____

Procedure_____ Date_____
Doctor_____ Ph.# _____
Where was procedure performed?_____
Reason for procedure_____

Adverse reaction during or after procedure _____

Was procedure successful? Y N   Procedure needed again? Y   N

Procedure ordered during Doctor visit listed on page _____

Procedure_____ Date_____
Doctor_____ Ph.# _____
Where was procedure performed?_____
Reason for procedure_____

Adverse reaction during or after procedure _____

Was procedure successful? Y N   Procedure needed again? Y   N

Procedure ordered during Doctor visit listed on page _____

Procedure_____ Date_____
Doctor_____ Ph.# _____
Where was procedure performed?_____
Reason for procedure_____

Adverse reaction during or after procedure _____

Was procedure successful? Y N   Procedure needed again? Y   N

Procedure ordered during Doctor visit listed on page _____

Procedure_____ Date_____

Doctor_____ Ph.#_____

Where was procedure performed?_____

Reason for procedure_____

Adverse reaction during or after procedure _____

Was procedure successful? Y N Procedure needed again? Y   N

Procedure ordered during Doctor visit listed on page _____

Procedure_____ Date_____

Doctor_____ Ph.#_____

Where was procedure performed?_____

Reason for procedure_____

Adverse reaction during or after procedure _____

Was procedure successful? Y N Procedure needed again? Y   N

Procedure ordered during Doctor visit listed on page _____

Procedure_____ Date_____

Doctor_____ Ph.#_____

Where was procedure performed?_____

Reason for procedure_____

Adverse reaction during or after procedure _____

Was procedure successful? Y N Procedure needed again? Y   N

Procedure ordered during Doctor visit listed on page _____

Procedure_____ Date_____

Doctor_____ Ph.# _____

Where was procedure performed?_____

Reason for procedure_____

Adverse reaction during or after procedure _____

Was procedure successful? Y N   Procedure needed again? Y   N

Procedure ordered during Doctor visit listed on page _____

Procedure_____ Date_____

Doctor_____ Ph.# _____

Where was procedure performed?_____

Reason for procedure_____

Adverse reaction during or after procedure _____

Was procedure successful? Y N   Procedure needed again? Y   N

Procedure ordered during Doctor visit listed on page _____

Procedure_____ Date_____

Doctor_____ Ph.# _____

Where was procedure performed?_____

Reason for procedure_____

Adverse reaction during or after procedure _____

Was procedure successful? Y N   Procedure needed again? Y   N

Procedure ordered during Doctor visit listed on page _____

Procedure_____ Date_____

Doctor_____ Ph.# _____

Where was procedure performed?_____

Reason for procedure_____

Adverse reaction during or after procedure _____

Was procedure successful? Y N Procedure needed again? Y N

Procedure ordered during Doctor visit listed on page _____

Procedure_____ Date_____

Doctor_____ Ph.# _____

Where was procedure performed?_____

Reason for procedure_____

Adverse reaction during or after procedure _____

Was procedure successful? Y N Procedure needed again? Y N

Procedure ordered during Doctor visit listed on page _____

Procedure_____ Date_____

Doctor_____ Ph.# _____

Where was procedure performed?_____

Reason for procedure_____

Adverse reaction during or after procedure _____

Was procedure successful? Y N Procedure needed again? Y N

Procedure ordered during Doctor visit listed on page _____

Procedure_____ Date_____

Doctor_____ Ph.# _____

Where was procedure performed?_____

Reason for procedure_____

Adverse reaction during or after procedure _____

Was procedure successful? Y N Procedure needed again? Y N

Procedure ordered during Doctor visit listed on page _____

Procedure_____ Date_____

Doctor_____ Ph.# _____

Where was procedure performed?_____

Reason for procedure_____

Adverse reaction during or after procedure _____

Was procedure successful? Y N Procedure needed again? Y N

Procedure ordered during Doctor visit listed on page _____

Procedure_____ Date_____

Doctor_____ Ph.# _____

Where was procedure performed?_____

Reason for procedure_____

Adverse reaction during or after procedure _____

Was procedure successful? Y N Procedure needed again? Y N

Procedure ordered during Doctor visit listed on page _____

Procedure_____ Date_____
Doctor_____Ph.# _____
Where was procedure performed?_____
Reason for procedure_____

Adverse reaction during or after procedure _____

Was procedure successful? Y N Procedure needed again? Y N

Procedure ordered during Doctor visit listed on page _____

Procedure_____ Date_____
Doctor_____Ph.# _____
Where was procedure performed?_____
Reason for procedure_____

Adverse reaction during or after procedure _____

Was procedure successful? Y N Procedure needed again? Y N

Procedure ordered during Doctor visit listed on page _____

Procedure_____ Date_____
Doctor_____Ph.# _____
Where was procedure performed?_____
Reason for procedure_____

Adverse reaction during or after procedure _____

Was procedure successful? Y N Procedure needed again? Y N

Procedure ordered during Doctor visit listed on page _____

Surgeries

In early Asian civilizations, the practice of medicine by physicians was particularly advanced for the time, with surgical techniques in India including the removal of tumors, bladder stones, and even cataracts.
https://www.factretriever.com/doctor-facts

Surgery _____ Date_____

Surgeon _____ Ph.# _____

Where was surgery performed?   _____

Reason for surgery_____

_____

Adverse reaction during or after surgery _____

_____

Length of hospital stay after surgery_____

Length of recovery from surgery _____

Was surgery successful? _____

Surgery ordered during Doctor visit listed on page _____

Surgery _____ Date_____

Surgeon _____ Ph.# _____

Where was surgery performed?   _____

Reason for surgery_____

_____

Adverse reaction during or after surgery _____

_____

Length of hospital stay after surgery_____

Length of recovery from surgery _____

Was surgery successful? _____

Surgery ordered during Doctor visit listed on page _____

Surgery _____ Date_____

Surgeon _____ Ph.# _____

Where was surgery performed? _____

Reason for surgery_____

_____

_____

Adverse reaction during or after surgery _____

_____

Length of hospital stay after surgery_____

Length of recovery from surgery _____

Was surgery successful? _____

Surgery ordered during Doctor visit listed on page _____

Surgery _____ Date_____

Surgeon _____ Ph.# _____

Where was surgery performed? _____

Reason for surgery_____

_____

_____

Adverse reaction during or after surgery _____

_____

Length of hospital stay after surgery_____

Length of recovery from surgery _____

Was surgery successful? _____

Surgery ordered during Doctor visit listed on page _____

Surgery _____ Date_____

Surgeon _____ Ph.# _____

Where was surgery performed? _____

Reason for surgery_____

Adverse reaction during or after surgery _____

Length of hospital stay after surgery_____

Length of recovery from surgery _____

Was surgery successful? _____

Surgery ordered during Doctor visit listed on page _____

Surgery _____ Date_____

Surgeon _____ Ph.# _____

Where was surgery performed? _____

Reason for surgery_____

Adverse reaction during or after surgery _____

Length of hospital stay after surgery_____

Length of recovery from surgery _____

Was surgery successful? _____

Surgery ordered during Doctor visit listed on page _____

Surgery _____ Date_____

Surgeon _____ Ph.# _____

Where was surgery performed? _____

Reason for surgery_____

Adverse reaction during or after surgery _____

Length of hospital stay after surgery_____

Length of recovery from surgery _____

Was surgery successful? _____

Surgery ordered during Doctor visit listed on page _____

Surgery _____ Date_____

Surgeon _____ Ph.# _____

Where was surgery performed? _____

Reason for surgery_____

Adverse reaction during or after surgery _____

Length of hospital stay after surgery_____

Length of recovery from surgery _____

Was surgery successful? _____

Surgery ordered during Doctor visit listed on page _____

Surgery _____ Date_____

Surgeon _____ Ph.# _____

Where was surgery performed? _____

Reason for surgery_____

Adverse reaction during or after surgery _____

Length of hospital stay after surgery_____

Length of recovery from surgery _____

Was surgery successful? _____

Surgery ordered during Doctor visit listed on page ____

Surgery _____ Date_____

Surgeon _____ Ph.# _____

Where was surgery performed? _____

Reason for surgery_____

Adverse reaction during or after surgery _____

Length of hospital stay after surgery_____

Length of recovery from surgery _____

Was surgery successful? _____

Surgery ordered during Doctor visit listed on page ____

Surgery _____ Date_____

Surgeon _____ Ph.# _____

Where was surgery performed? _____

Reason for surgery_____

Adverse reaction during or after surgery _____

Length of hospital stay after surgery_____

Length of recovery from surgery _____

Was surgery successful? _____

Surgery ordered during Doctor visit listed on page _____

Surgery _____ Date_____

Surgeon _____ Ph.# _____

Where was surgery performed? _____

Reason for surgery_____

Adverse reaction during or after surgery _____

Length of hospital stay after surgery_____

Length of recovery from surgery _____

Was surgery successful? _____

Surgery ordered during Doctor visit listed on page _____

Surgery _____ Date_____

Surgeon _____ Ph.# _____

Where was surgery performed? _____

Reason for surgery_____

Adverse reaction during or after surgery _____

Length of hospital stay after surgery_____

Length of recovery from surgery _____

Was surgery successful? _____

Surgery ordered during Doctor visit listed on page _____

Surgery _____ Date_____

Surgeon _____ Ph.# _____

Where was surgery performed? _____

Reason for surgery_____

Adverse reaction during or after surgery _____

Length of hospital stay after surgery_____

Length of recovery from surgery _____

Was surgery successful? _____

Surgery ordered during Doctor visit listed on page _____

Surgery _____ Date_____

Surgeon _____ Ph.# _____

Where was surgery performed? _____

Reason for surgery_____

_____

Adverse reaction during or after surgery _____

_____

Length of hospital stay after surgery_____

Length of recovery from surgery _____

Was surgery successful? _____

Surgery ordered during Doctor visit listed on page _____

Surgery _____ Date_____

Surgeon _____ Ph.# _____

Where was surgery performed? _____

Reason for surgery_____

_____

Adverse reaction during or after surgery _____

_____

Length of hospital stay after surgery_____

Length of recovery from surgery _____

Was surgery successful? _____

Surgery ordered during Doctor visit listed on page _____

Surgery _____ Date_____

Surgeon _____ Ph.# _____

Where was surgery performed? _____

Reason for surgery_____

Adverse reaction during or after surgery _____

Length of hospital stay after surgery_____

Length of recovery from surgery _____

Was surgery successful? _____

Surgery ordered during Doctor visit listed on page _____

Surgery _____ Date_____

Surgeon _____ Ph.# _____

Where was surgery performed? _____

Reason for surgery_____

Adverse reaction during or after surgery _____

Length of hospital stay after surgery_____

Length of recovery from surgery _____

Was surgery successful? _____

Surgery ordered during Doctor visit listed on page _____

Surgery _____ Date_____

Surgeon _____ Ph.# _____

Where was surgery performed? _____

Reason for surgery_____

_____

Adverse reaction during or after surgery _____

_____

Length of hospital stay after surgery_____

Length of recovery from surgery _____

Was surgery successful? _____

Surgery ordered during Doctor visit listed on page _____

Surgery _____ Date_____

Surgeon _____ Ph.# _____

Where was surgery performed? _____

Reason for surgery_____

_____

Adverse reaction during or after surgery _____

_____

Length of hospital stay after surgery_____

Length of recovery from surgery _____

Was surgery successful? _____

Surgery ordered during Doctor visit listed on page _____

Blood Work

What is blood made of?

The components of human blood include:

***Plasma.** This is the liquid part of blood. The following
        blood cells are suspended in plasma:

***Red Blood cells (erythrocytes).**
        These carry oxygen from the lungs to the rest of the body.

***White Blood cells (leukocytes).**
        These help fight infections and aid in the immune process.

Platelets (thrombocytes).
        These help to control bleeding.

https://www.hopkinsmedicine.org/health/wellness-and-prevention/facts-about-blood

---

Blood drawn at _____ Date_____

Date Blood work results reviewed or seen by you _____

Blood levels that were out of normal range_____

Blood work ordered during Doctor visit listed on page_____

Blood drawn at _____ Date_____

Date Blood work results reviewed or seen by you _____

Blood levels that were out of normal range_____

Blood work ordered during Doctor visit listed on page_____

Blood drawn at _____ Date_____

Date Blood work results reviewed or seen by you _____

Blood levels that were out of normal range_____

Blood work ordered during Doctor visit listed on page_____

Blood drawn at _____ Date_____

Date Blood work results reviewed or seen by you _____

Blood levels that were out of normal range_____

Blood work ordered during Doctor visit listed on page_____

Blood drawn at _____ Date_____

Date Blood work results reviewed or seen by you _____

Blood levels that were out of normal range_____

_____

Blood work ordered during Doctor visit listed on page_____

Blood drawn at _____ Date_____

Date Blood work results reviewed or seen by you _____

Blood levels that were out of normal range_____

_____

Blood work ordered during Doctor visit listed on page_____

Blood drawn at _____ Date_____

Date Blood work results reviewed or seen by you _____

Blood levels that were out of normal range_____

_____

Blood work ordered during Doctor visit listed on page_____

Blood drawn at _____ Date_____

Date Blood work results reviewed or seen by you _____

Blood levels that were out of normal range_____

_____

Blood work ordered during Doctor visit listed on page_____

Blood drawn at _____ Date_____

Date Blood work results reviewed or seen by you _____

Blood levels that were out of normal range_____

Blood work ordered during Doctor visit listed on page_____

Blood drawn at _____ Date_____

Date Blood work results reviewed or seen by you _____

Blood levels that were out of normal range_____

Blood work ordered during Doctor visit listed on page_____

Blood drawn at _____ Date_____

Date Blood work results reviewed or seen by you _____

Blood levels that were out of normal range_____

Blood work ordered during Doctor visit listed on page_____

Blood drawn at _____ Date_____

Date Blood work results reviewed or seen by you _____

Blood levels that were out of normal range_____

Blood work ordered during Doctor visit listed on page_____

Blood drawn at _____ Date_____

Date Blood work results reviewed or seen by you _____

Blood levels that were out of normal range_____

_____

Blood work ordered during Doctor visit listed on page_____

Blood drawn at _____ Date_____

Date Blood work results reviewed or seen by you _____

Blood levels that were out of normal range_____

_____

Blood work ordered during Doctor visit listed on page_____

Blood drawn at _____ Date_____

Date Blood work results reviewed or seen by you _____

Blood levels that were out of normal range_____

_____

Blood work ordered during Doctor visit listed on page_____

Blood drawn at _____ Date_____

Date Blood work results reviewed or seen by you _____

Blood levels that were out of normal range_____

_____

Blood work ordered during Doctor visit listed on page_____

Blood drawn at _____ Date_____
Date Blood work results reviewed or seen by you _____
Blood levels that were out of normal range_____

Blood work ordered during Doctor visit listed on page_____

Blood drawn at _____ Date_____
Date Blood work results reviewed or seen by you _____
Blood levels that were out of normal range_____

Blood work ordered during Doctor visit listed on page_____

Blood drawn at _____ Date_____
Date Blood work results reviewed or seen by you _____
Blood levels that were out of normal range_____

Blood work ordered during Doctor visit listed on page_____

Blood drawn at _____ Date_____
Date Blood work results reviewed or seen by you _____
Blood levels that were out of normal range_____

Blood work ordered during Doctor visit listed on page_____

Blood drawn at _____ Date_____

Date Blood work results reviewed or seen by you _____

Blood levels that were out of normal range_____

_____

Blood work ordered during Doctor visit listed on page_____

Blood drawn at _____ Date_____

Date Blood work results reviewed or seen by you _____

Blood levels that were out of normal range_____

_____

Blood work ordered during Doctor visit listed on page_____

Blood drawn at _____ Date_____

Date Blood work results reviewed or seen by you _____

Blood levels that were out of normal range_____

_____

Blood work ordered during Doctor visit listed on page_____

Blood drawn at _____ Date_____

Date Blood work results reviewed or seen by you _____

Blood levels that were out of normal range_____

_____

Blood work ordered during Doctor visit listed on page_____

Blood drawn at _____ Date_____

Date Blood work results reviewed or seen by you _____

Blood levels that were out of normal range_____

Blood work ordered during Doctor visit listed on page_____

Blood drawn at _____ Date_____

Date Blood work results reviewed or seen by you _____

Blood levels that were out of normal range_____

Blood work ordered during Doctor visit listed on page_____

Blood drawn at _____ Date_____

Date Blood work results reviewed or seen by you _____

Blood levels that were out of normal range_____

Blood work ordered during Doctor visit listed on page_____

Blood drawn at _____ Date_____

Date Blood work results reviewed or seen by you _____

Blood levels that were out of normal range_____

Blood work ordered during Doctor visit listed on page_____

Blood drawn at _____ Date_____

Date Blood work results reviewed or seen by you _____

Blood levels that were out of normal range_____

_____

Blood work ordered during Doctor visit listed on page_____

Blood drawn at _____ Date_____

Date Blood work results reviewed or seen by you _____

Blood levels that were out of normal range_____

_____

Blood work ordered during Doctor visit listed on page_____

Blood drawn at _____ Date_____

Date Blood work results reviewed or seen by you _____

Blood levels that were out of normal range_____

_____

Blood work ordered during Doctor visit listed on page_____

Blood drawn at _____ Date_____

Date Blood work results reviewed or seen by you _____

Blood levels that were out of normal range_____

_____

Blood work ordered during Doctor visit listed on page_____

Blood drawn at _____ Date_____

Date Blood work results reviewed or seen by you _____

Blood levels that were out of normal range_____

Blood work ordered during Doctor visit listed on page_____

Blood drawn at _____ Date_____

Date Blood work results reviewed or seen by you _____

Blood levels that were out of normal range_____

Blood work ordered during Doctor visit listed on page_____

Blood drawn at _____ Date_____

Date Blood work results reviewed or seen by you _____

Blood levels that were out of normal range_____

Blood work ordered during Doctor visit listed on page_____

Blood drawn at _____ Date_____

Date Blood work results reviewed or seen by you _____

Blood levels that were out of normal range_____

Blood work ordered during Doctor visit listed on page_____

Blood drawn at _____ Date_____

Date Blood work results reviewed or seen by you _____

Blood levels that were out of normal range_____

_____

Blood work ordered during Doctor visit listed on page_____

Blood drawn at _____ Date_____

Date Blood work results reviewed or seen by you _____

Blood levels that were out of normal range_____

_____

Blood work ordered during Doctor visit listed on page_____

Blood drawn at _____ Date_____

Date Blood work results reviewed or seen by you _____

Blood levels that were out of normal range_____

_____

Blood work ordered during Doctor visit listed on page_____

Blood drawn at _____ Date_____

Date Blood work results reviewed or seen by you _____

Blood levels that were out of normal range_____

_____

Blood work ordered during Doctor visit listed on page_____

Blood drawn at _____ Date_____
Date Blood work results reviewed or seen by you _____
Blood levels that were out of normal range_____

Blood work ordered during Doctor visit listed on page_____

Blood drawn at _____ Date_____
Date Blood work results reviewed or seen by you _____
Blood levels that were out of normal range_____

Blood work ordered during Doctor visit listed on page_____

Blood drawn at _____ Date_____
Date Blood work results reviewed or seen by you _____
Blood levels that were out of normal range_____

Blood work ordered during Doctor visit listed on page_____

Blood drawn at _____ Date_____
Date Blood work results reviewed or seen by you _____
Blood levels that were out of normal range_____

Blood work ordered during Doctor visit listed on page_____

Blood drawn at _____ Date_____

Date Blood work results reviewed or seen by you _____

Blood levels that were out of normal range_____

_____

Blood work ordered during Doctor visit listed on page_____

Blood drawn at _____ Date_____

Date Blood work results reviewed or seen by you _____

Blood levels that were out of normal range_____

_____

Blood work ordered during Doctor visit listed on page_____

Blood drawn at _____ Date_____

Date Blood work results reviewed or seen by you _____

Blood levels that were out of normal range_____

_____

Blood work ordered during Doctor visit listed on page_____

Blood drawn at _____ Date_____

Date Blood work results reviewed or seen by you _____

Blood levels that were out of normal range_____

_____

Blood work ordered during Doctor visit listed on page_____

Blood drawn at _____ Date_____

Date Blood work results reviewed or seen by you _____

Blood levels that were out of normal range_____

Blood work ordered during Doctor visit listed on page_____

Blood drawn at _____ Date_____

Date Blood work results reviewed or seen by you _____

Blood levels that were out of normal range_____

Blood work ordered during Doctor visit listed on page_____

Blood drawn at _____ Date_____

Date Blood work results reviewed or seen by you _____

Blood levels that were out of normal range_____

Blood work ordered during Doctor visit listed on page_____

Blood drawn at _____ Date_____

Date Blood work results reviewed or seen by you _____

Blood levels that were out of normal range_____

Blood work ordered during Doctor visit listed on page_____

Blood drawn at _____ Date_____

Date Blood work results reviewed or seen by you _____

Blood levels that were out of normal range_____

_____

Blood work ordered during Doctor visit listed on page_____

Blood drawn at _____ Date_____

Date Blood work results reviewed or seen by you _____

Blood levels that were out of normal range_____

_____

Blood work ordered during Doctor visit listed on page_____

Blood drawn at _____ Date_____

Date Blood work results reviewed or seen by you _____

Blood levels that were out of normal range_____

_____

Blood work ordered during Doctor visit listed on page_____

Blood drawn at _____ Date_____

Date Blood work results reviewed or seen by you _____

Blood levels that were out of normal range_____

_____

Blood work ordered during Doctor visit listed on page_____

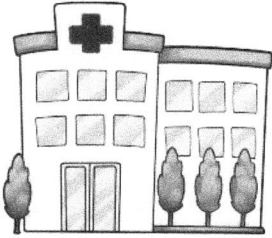

Hospital Stays

The national average for a hospital stay is **4.5 days**, according to the Agency for Healthcare Research and Quality, at an average cost of $10,400 per day.

Hospital_____

Address_____

Date and duration of stay _____

Reason for stay_____

This stay associated with surgery or doctor visit on page_____

Hospital_____

Address_____

Date and duration of stay _____

Reason for stay_____

This stay associated with surgery or doctor visit on page_____

Hospital_____

Address_____

Date and duration of stay _____

Reason for stay_____

This stay associated with surgery or doctor visit on page_____

Hospital_____

Address_____

Date and duration of stay _____

Reason for stay_____

This stay associated with surgery or doctor visit on page_____

Hospital_____

Address_____

Date and duration of stay _____

Reason for stay_____

This stay associated with surgery or doctor visit on page_____

Hospital_____

Address_____

Date and duration of stay _____

Reason for stay_____

This stay associated with surgery or doctor visit on page_____

Hospital_____

Address_____

Date and duration of stay _____

Reason for stay_____

This stay associated with surgery or doctor visit on page_____

Hospital_____

Address_____

Date and duration of stay _____

Reason for stay_____

This stay associated with surgery or doctor visit on page_____

Hospital_____

Address_____

Date and duration of stay _____

Reason for stay_____

This stay associated with surgery or doctor visit on page_____

Hospital_____

Address_____

Date and duration of stay _____

Reason for stay_____

This stay associated with surgery or doctor visit on page_____

Hospital_____

Address_____

Date and duration of stay _____

Reason for stay_____

This stay associated with surgery or doctor visit on page_____

Hospital_____

Address_____

Date and duration of stay _____

Reason for stay_____

This stay associated with surgery or doctor visit on page_____

Hospital_____

Address_____

Date and duration of stay _____

Reason for stay_____

This stay associated with surgery or doctor visit on page_____

Hospital_____

Address_____

Date and duration of stay _____

Reason for stay_____

This stay associated with surgery or doctor visit on page_____

Hospital_____

Address_____

Date and duration of stay _____

Reason for stay_____

This stay associated with surgery or doctor visit on page_____

Hospital_____

Address_____

Date and duration of stay _____

Reason for stay_____

This stay associated with surgery or doctor visit on page_____

Hospital_____

Address_____

Date and duration of stay _____

Reason for stay_____

This stay associated with surgery or doctor visit on page_____

Hospital_____

Address_____

Date and duration of stay _____

Reason for stay_____

This stay associated with surgery or doctor visit on page_____

Hospital_____

Address_____

Date and duration of stay _____

Reason for stay_____

This stay associated with surgery or doctor visit on page_____

Hospital_____

Address_____

Date and duration of stay _____

Reason for stay_____

This stay associated with surgery or doctor visit on page_____

Hospital_____

Address_____

Date and duration of stay _____

Reason for stay_____

This stay associated with surgery or doctor visit on page_____

Hospital_____

Address_____

Date and duration of stay _____

Reason for stay_____

This stay associated with surgery or doctor visit on page_____

Hospital_____

Address_____

Date and duration of stay _____

Reason for stay_____

This stay associated with surgery or doctor visit on page_____

Hospital_____

Address_____

Date and duration of stay _____

Reason for stay_____

This stay associated with surgery or doctor visit on page_____

Hospital_____

Address_____

Date and duration of stay _____

Reason for stay_____

This stay associated with surgery or doctor visit on page_____

Hospital_____

Address_____

Date and duration of stay _____

Reason for stay_____

This stay associated with surgery or doctor visit on page_____

Hospital_____

Address_____

Date and duration of stay _____

Reason for stay_____

This stay associated with surgery or doctor visit on page_____

Hospital_____

Address_____

Date and duration of stay _____

Reason for stay_____

This stay associated with surgery or doctor visit on page_____

Hospital_____

Address_____

Date and duration of stay _____

Reason for stay_____

This stay associated with surgery or doctor visit on page_____

Hospital_____

Address_____

Date and duration of stay _____

Reason for stay_____

This stay associated with surgery or doctor visit on page_____

Hospital_____

Address_____

Date and duration of stay _____

Reason for stay_____

This stay associated with surgery or doctor visit on page_____

Hospital_____

Address_____

Date and duration of stay _____

Reason for stay_____

This stay associated with surgery or doctor visit on page_____

DENTAL

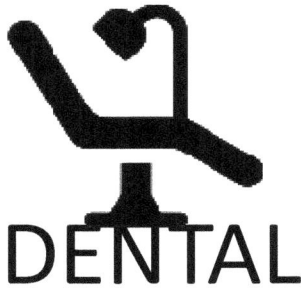

Cleanings, Check-ups, Fillings

The very first dentist ever is considered to be Hesy-Re, who practiced around 2600 B.C. He was also an Egyptian scribe. We know he was what we would consider a dentist, thanks to the inscription on his tomb. It read, "the greatest of those who deal with teeth and of physicians."
https://atooth.com

Dentist_____ Date _____

Dentist Address _____ Ph# _____

Was this appointment a regular check-up? Y N With x-rays? Y N

Was this appointment for a cleaning? Y N   For a filling? Y N

For a root canal? Y N   For a cap? Y N   For an extraction? Y N

Which tooth (teeth) was treated? _____

Results of check-up and x-rays_____

Treatment plan _____

Dentist_____ Date _____

Dentist Address _____ Ph# _____

Was this appointment a regular check-up? Y N With x-rays? Y N

Was this appointment for a cleaning? Y N   For a filling? Y N

For a root canal? Y N   For a cap? Y N   For an extraction? Y N

Which tooth (teeth) was treated? _____

Results of check-up and x-rays_____

Treatment plan _____

Dentist_____ Date _____

Dentist Address _____ Ph# _____

Was this appointment a regular check-up? Y N With x-rays? Y N

Was this appointment for a cleaning? Y N   For a filling? Y N

For a root canal? Y N   For a cap? Y N   For an extraction? Y N

Which tooth (teeth) was treated? _____

Results of check-up and x-rays_____

Treatment plan _____

Dentist_____ Date _____

Dentist Address _____ Ph#_____

Was this appointment a regular check-up? Y N With x-rays? Y N

Was this appointment for a cleaning? Y N   For a filling? Y N

For a root canal? Y N   For a cap? Y N   For an extraction? Y N

Which tooth (teeth) was treated? _____

Results of check-up and x-rays_____

_____

Treatment plan _____

Dentist_____ Date _____

Dentist Address _____ Ph#_____

Was this appointment a regular check-up? Y N With x-rays? Y N

Was this appointment for a cleaning? Y N   For a filling? Y N

For a root canal? Y N   For a cap? Y N   For an extraction? Y N

Which tooth (teeth) was treated? _____

Results of check-up and x-rays_____

_____

Treatment plan _____

Dentist_____ Date _____

Dentist Address _____ Ph#_____

Was this appointment a regular check-up? Y N With x-rays? Y N

Was this appointment for a cleaning? Y N   For a filling? Y N

For a root canal? Y N   For a cap? Y N   For an extraction? Y N

Which tooth (teeth) was treated? _____

Results of check-up and x-rays_____

_____

Treatment plan _____

Dentist_____ Date _____

Dentist Address _____ Ph# _____

Was this appointment a regular check-up? Y N With x-rays? Y N

Was this appointment for a cleaning? Y N   For a filling? Y N

For a root canal? Y N   For a cap? Y N   For an extraction? Y N

Which tooth (teeth) was treated? _____

Results of check-up and x-rays_____

Treatment plan _____

Dentist_____ Date _____

Dentist Address _____ Ph# _____

Was this appointment a regular check-up? Y N With x-rays? Y N

Was this appointment for a cleaning? Y N   For a filling? Y N

For a root canal? Y N   For a cap? Y N   For an extraction? Y N

Which tooth (teeth) was treated? _____

Results of check-up and x-rays_____

Treatment plan _____

Dentist_____ Date _____

Dentist Address _____ Ph# _____

Was this appointment a regular check-up? Y N With x-rays? Y N

Was this appointment for a cleaning? Y N   For a filling? Y N

For a root canal? Y N   For a cap? Y N   For an extraction? Y N

Which tooth (teeth) was treated? _____

Results of check-up and x-rays_____

Treatment plan _____

Dentist_____ Date _____

Dentist Address _____ Ph# _____

Was this appointment a regular check-up? Y N With x-rays? Y N

Was this appointment for a cleaning? Y N   For a filling? Y N

For a root canal? Y N   For a cap? Y N   For an extraction? Y N

Which tooth (teeth) was treated? _____

Results of check-up and x-rays_____

Treatment plan _____

Dentist_____ Date _____

Dentist Address _____ Ph# _____

Was this appointment a regular check-up? Y N With x-rays? Y N

Was this appointment for a cleaning? Y N   For a filling? Y N

For a root canal? Y N   For a cap? Y N   For an extraction? Y N

Which tooth (teeth) was treated? _____

Results of check-up and x-rays_____

Treatment plan _____

Dentist_____ Date _____

Dentist Address _____ Ph# _____

Was this appointment a regular check-up? Y N With x-rays? Y N

Was this appointment for a cleaning? Y N   For a filling? Y N

For a root canal? Y N   For a cap? Y N   For an extraction? Y N

Which tooth (teeth) was treated? _____

Results of check-up and x-rays_____

Treatment plan _____

Dentist_____ Date _____

Dentist Address _____ Ph# _____

Was this appointment a regular check-up? Y N With x-rays? Y N

Was this appointment for a cleaning? Y N   For a filling? Y N

For a root canal? Y N   For a cap? Y N   For an extraction? Y N

Which tooth (teeth) was treated? _____

Results of check-up and x-rays_____

Treatment plan _____

Dentist_____ Date _____

Dentist Address _____ Ph# _____

Was this appointment a regular check-up? Y N With x-rays? Y N

Was this appointment for a cleaning? Y N   For a filling? Y N

For a root canal? Y N   For a cap? Y N   For an extraction? Y N

Which tooth (teeth) was treated? _____

Results of check-up and x-rays_____

Treatment plan _____

Dentist_____ Date _____

Dentist Address _____ Ph# _____

Was this appointment a regular check-up? Y N With x-rays? Y N

Was this appointment for a cleaning? Y N   For a filling? Y N

For a root canal? Y N   For a cap? Y N   For an extraction? Y N

Which tooth (teeth) was treated? _____

Results of check-up and x-rays_____

Treatment plan _____

Dentist_____ Date _____

Dentist Address _____ Ph# _____

Was this appointment a regular check-up? Y N With x-rays? Y N

Was this appointment for a cleaning? Y N   For a filling? Y N

For a root canal? Y N   For a cap? Y N   For an extraction? Y N

Which tooth (teeth) was treated? _____

Results of check-up and x-rays_____

Treatment plan _____

Dentist_____ Date _____

Dentist Address _____ Ph# _____

Was this appointment a regular check-up? Y N With x-rays? Y N

Was this appointment for a cleaning? Y N   For a filling? Y N

For a root canal? Y N   For a cap? Y N   For an extraction? Y N

Which tooth (teeth) was treated? _____

Results of check-up and x-rays_____

Treatment plan _____

Dentist_____ Date _____

Dentist Address _____ Ph# _____

Was this appointment a regular check-up? Y N With x-rays? Y N

Was this appointment for a cleaning? Y N   For a filling? Y N

For a root canal? Y N   For a cap? Y N   For an extraction? Y N

Which tooth (teeth) was treated? _____

Results of check-up and x-rays_____

Treatment plan _____

Dentist_____ Date _____

Dentist Address _____ Ph# _____

Was this appointment a regular check-up? Y N With x-rays? Y N

Was this appointment for a cleaning? Y N   For a filling? Y N

For a root canal? Y N   For a cap? Y N   For an extraction? Y N

Which tooth (teeth) was treated? _____

Results of check-up and x-rays_____

_____

Treatment plan _____

Dentist_____ Date _____

Dentist Address _____ Ph# _____

Was this appointment a regular check-up? Y N With x-rays? Y N

Was this appointment for a cleaning? Y N   For a filling? Y N

For a root canal? Y N   For a cap? Y N   For an extraction? Y N

Which tooth (teeth) was treated? _____

Results of check-up and x-rays_____

_____

Treatment plan _____

Dentist_____ Date _____

Dentist Address _____ Ph# _____

Was this appointment a regular check-up? Y N With x-rays? Y N

Was this appointment for a cleaning? Y N   For a filling? Y N

For a root canal? Y N   For a cap? Y N   For an extraction? Y N

Which tooth (teeth) was treated? _____

Results of check-up and x-rays_____

_____

Treatment plan _____

Dentist _____ Date _____

Dentist Address _____ Ph# _____

Was this appointment a regular check-up? Y N With x-rays? Y N

Was this appointment for a cleaning? Y N   For a filling? Y N

For a root canal? Y N   For a cap? Y N   For an extraction? Y N

Which tooth (teeth) was treated? _____

Results of check-up and x-rays_____

Treatment plan _____

Dentist _____ Date _____

Dentist Address _____ Ph# _____

Was this appointment a regular check-up? Y N With x-rays? Y N

Was this appointment for a cleaning? Y N   For a filling? Y N

For a root canal? Y N   For a cap? Y N   For an extraction? Y N

Which tooth (teeth) was treated? _____

Results of check-up and x-rays_____

Treatment plan _____

Dentist _____ Date _____

Dentist Address _____ Ph# _____

Was this appointment a regular check-up? Y N With x-rays? Y N

Was this appointment for a cleaning? Y N   For a filling? Y N

For a root canal? Y N   For a cap? Y N   For an extraction? Y N

Which tooth (teeth) was treated? _____

Results of check-up and x-rays_____

Treatment plan _____

Dentist_____ Date _____

Dentist Address _____ Ph# _____

Was this appointment a regular check-up? Y N With x-rays? Y N

Was this appointment for a cleaning? Y N   For a filling? Y N

For a root canal? Y N   For a cap? Y N   For an extraction? Y N

Which tooth (teeth) was treated? _____

Results of check-up and x-rays_____

Treatment plan _____

Dentist_____ Date _____

Dentist Address _____ Ph# _____

Was this appointment a regular check-up? Y N With x-rays? Y N

Was this appointment for a cleaning? Y N   For a filling? Y N

For a root canal? Y N   For a cap? Y N   For an extraction? Y N

Which tooth (teeth) was treated? _____

Results of check-up and x-rays_____

Treatment plan _____

Dentist_____ Date _____

Dentist Address _____ Ph# _____

Was this appointment a regular check-up? Y N With x-rays? Y N

Was this appointment for a cleaning? Y N   For a filling? Y N

For a root canal? Y N   For a cap? Y N   For an extraction? Y N

Which tooth (teeth) was treated? _____

Results of check-up and x-rays_____

Treatment plan _____

Dentist_____ Date _____

Dentist Address _____ Ph# _____

Was this appointment a regular check-up? Y N With x-rays? Y N

Was this appointment for a cleaning? Y N   For a filling? Y N

For a root canal? Y N   For a cap? Y N   For an extraction? Y N

Which tooth (teeth) was treated? _____

Results of check-up and x-rays_____

Treatment plan _____

Dentist_____ Date _____

Dentist Address _____ Ph# _____

Was this appointment a regular check-up? Y N With x-rays? Y N

Was this appointment for a cleaning? Y N   For a filling? Y N

For a root canal? Y N   For a cap? Y N   For an extraction? Y N

Which tooth (teeth) was treated? _____

Results of check-up and x-rays_____

Treatment plan _____

Dentist_____ Date _____

Dentist Address _____ Ph# _____

Was this appointment a regular check-up? Y N With x-rays? Y N

Was this appointment for a cleaning? Y N   For a filling? Y N

For a root canal? Y N   For a cap? Y N   For an extraction? Y N

Which tooth (teeth) was treated? _____

Results of check-up and x-rays_____

Treatment plan _____

Dentist_____ Date _____

Dentist Address _____ Ph# _____

Was this appointment a regular check-up? Y N With x-rays? Y N

Was this appointment for a cleaning? Y N   For a filling? Y N

For a root canal? Y N   For a cap? Y N   For an extraction? Y N

Which tooth (teeth) was treated? _____

Results of check-up and x-rays_____

Treatment plan _____

Dentist_____ Date _____

Dentist Address _____ Ph# _____

Was this appointment a regular check-up? Y N With x-rays? Y N

Was this appointment for a cleaning? Y N   For a filling? Y N

For a root canal? Y N   For a cap? Y N   For an extraction? Y N

Which tooth (teeth) was treated? _____

Results of check-up and x-rays_____

Treatment plan _____

Dentist_____ Date _____

Dentist Address _____ Ph# _____

Was this appointment a regular check-up? Y N With x-rays? Y N

Was this appointment for a cleaning? Y N   For a filling? Y N

For a root canal? Y N   For a cap? Y N   For an extraction? Y N

Which tooth (teeth) was treated? _____

Results of check-up and x-rays_____

Treatment plan _____

Dentist_____ Date _____

Dentist Address _____ Ph#_____

Was this appointment a regular check-up? Y N With x-rays? Y N

Was this appointment for a cleaning? Y N   For a filling? Y N

For a root canal? Y N   For a cap? Y N   For an extraction? Y N

Which tooth (teeth) was treated? _____

Results of check-up and x-rays_____

Treatment plan _____

Dentist_____ Date _____

Dentist Address _____ Ph#_____

Was this appointment a regular check-up? Y N With x-rays? Y N

Was this appointment for a cleaning? Y N   For a filling? Y N

For a root canal? Y N   For a cap? Y N   For an extraction? Y N

Which tooth (teeth) was treated? _____

Results of check-up and x-rays_____

Treatment plan _____

Dentist_____ Date _____

Dentist Address _____ Ph#_____

Was this appointment a regular check-up? Y N With x-rays? Y N

Was this appointment for a cleaning? Y N   For a filling? Y N

For a root canal? Y N   For a cap? Y N   For an extraction? Y N

Which tooth (teeth) was treated? _____

Results of check-up and x-rays_____

Treatment plan _____

Dentist_____ Date _____

Dentist Address _____ Ph# _____

Was this appointment a regular check-up? Y N With x-rays? Y N

Was this appointment for a cleaning? Y N   For a filling? Y N

For a root canal? Y N   For a cap? Y N   For an extraction? Y N

Which tooth (teeth) was treated? _____

Results of check-up and x-rays_____

_____

Treatment plan _____

Dentist_____ Date _____

Dentist Address _____ Ph# _____

Was this appointment a regular check-up? Y N With x-rays? Y N

Was this appointment for a cleaning? Y N   For a filling? Y N

For a root canal? Y N   For a cap? Y N   For an extraction? Y N

Which tooth (teeth) was treated? _____

Results of check-up and x-rays_____

_____

Treatment plan _____

Dentist_____ Date _____

Dentist Address _____ Ph# _____

Was this appointment a regular check-up? Y N With x-rays? Y N

Was this appointment for a cleaning? Y N   For a filling? Y N

For a root canal? Y N   For a cap? Y N   For an extraction? Y N

Which tooth (teeth) was treated? _____

Results of check-up and x-rays_____

_____

Treatment plan _____

Dentist_____ Date _____

Dentist Address _____ Ph#_____

Was this appointment a regular check-up? Y N With x-rays? Y N

Was this appointment for a cleaning? Y N   For a filling? Y N

For a root canal? Y N   For a cap? Y N   For an extraction? Y N

Which tooth (teeth) was treated? _____

Results of check-up and x-rays_____

Treatment plan _____

Dentist_____ Date _____

Dentist Address _____ Ph#_____

Was this appointment a regular check-up? Y N With x-rays? Y N

Was this appointment for a cleaning? Y N   For a filling? Y N

For a root canal? Y N   For a cap? Y N   For an extraction? Y N

Which tooth (teeth) was treated? _____

Results of check-up and x-rays_____

Treatment plan _____

Dentist_____ Date _____

Dentist Address _____ Ph#_____

Was this appointment a regular check-up? Y N With x-rays? Y N

Was this appointment for a cleaning? Y N   For a filling? Y N

For a root canal? Y N   For a cap? Y N   For an extraction? Y N

Which tooth (teeth) was treated? _____

Results of check-up and x-rays_____

Treatment plan _____

Dentist_____ Date _____

Dentist Address _____ Ph# _____

Was this appointment a regular check-up? Y N With x-rays? Y N

Was this appointment for a cleaning? Y N   For a filling? Y N

For a root canal? Y N   For a cap? Y N   For an extraction? Y N

Which tooth (teeth) was treated? _____

Results of check-up and x-rays_____

Treatment plan _____

Dentist_____ Date _____

Dentist Address _____ Ph# _____

Was this appointment a regular check-up? Y N With x-rays? Y N

Was this appointment for a cleaning? Y N   For a filling? Y N

For a root canal? Y N   For a cap? Y N   For an extraction? Y N

Which tooth (teeth) was treated? _____

Results of check-up and x-rays_____

Treatment plan _____

Dentist_____ Date _____

Dentist Address _____ Ph# _____

Was this appointment a regular check-up? Y N With x-rays? Y N

Was this appointment for a cleaning? Y N   For a filling? Y N

For a root canal? Y N   For a cap? Y N   For an extraction? Y N

Which tooth (teeth) was treated? _____

Results of check-up and x-rays_____

Treatment plan _____

Dentist_____ Date _____

Dentist Address _____ Ph#_____

Was this appointment a regular check-up? Y N With x-rays? Y N

Was this appointment for a cleaning? Y N   For a filling? Y N

For a root canal? Y N   For a cap? Y N   For an extraction? Y N

Which tooth (teeth) was treated? _____

Results of check-up and x-rays_____

Treatment plan _____

Dentist_____ Date _____

Dentist Address _____ Ph#_____

Was this appointment a regular check-up? Y N With x-rays? Y N

Was this appointment for a cleaning? Y N   For a filling? Y N

For a root canal? Y N   For a cap? Y N   For an extraction? Y N

Which tooth (teeth) was treated? _____

Results of check-up and x-rays_____

Treatment plan _____

Dentist_____ Date _____

Dentist Address _____ Ph#_____

Was this appointment a regular check-up? Y N With x-rays? Y N

Was this appointment for a cleaning? Y N   For a filling? Y N

For a root canal? Y N   For a cap? Y N   For an extraction? Y N

Which tooth (teeth) was treated? _____

Results of check-up and x-rays_____

Treatment plan _____

Dentist_____ Date _____

Dentist Address _____ Ph# _____

Was this appointment a regular check-up? Y N With x-rays? Y N

Was this appointment for a cleaning? Y N   For a filling? Y N

For a root canal? Y N   For a cap? Y N   For an extraction? Y N

Which tooth (teeth) was treated? _____

Results of check-up and x-rays_____

Treatment plan _____

Dentist_____ Date _____

Dentist Address _____ Ph# _____

Was this appointment a regular check-up? Y N With x-rays? Y N

Was this appointment for a cleaning? Y N   For a filling? Y N

For a root canal? Y N   For a cap? Y N   For an extraction? Y N

Which tooth (teeth) was treated? _____

Results of check-up and x-rays_____

Treatment plan _____

Dentist_____ Date _____

Dentist Address _____ Ph# _____

Was this appointment a regular check-up? Y N With x-rays? Y N

Was this appointment for a cleaning? Y N   For a filling? Y N

For a root canal? Y N   For a cap? Y N   For an extraction? Y N

Which tooth (teeth) was treated? _____

Results of check-up and x-rays_____

Treatment plan _____

Dentist_____ Date _____

Dentist Address _____ Ph# _____

Was this appointment a regular check-up? Y N With x-rays? Y N

Was this appointment for a cleaning? Y N   For a filling? Y N

For a root canal? Y N   For a cap? Y N   For an extraction? Y N

Which tooth (teeth) was treated? _____

Results of check-up and x-rays_____
_____

Treatment plan _____

Dentist_____ Date _____

Dentist Address _____ Ph# _____

Was this appointment a regular check-up? Y N With x-rays? Y N

Was this appointment for a cleaning? Y N   For a filling? Y N

For a root canal? Y N   For a cap? Y N   For an extraction? Y N

Which tooth (teeth) was treated? _____

Results of check-up and x-rays_____
_____

Treatment plan _____

Dentist_____ Date _____

Dentist Address _____ Ph# _____

Was this appointment a regular check-up? Y N With x-rays? Y N

Was this appointment for a cleaning? Y N   For a filling? Y N

For a root canal? Y N   For a cap? Y N   For an extraction? Y N

Which tooth (teeth) was treated? _____

Results of check-up and x-rays_____
_____

Treatment plan _____

Dentist_____ Date _____

Dentist Address _____ Ph# _____

Was this appointment a regular check-up? Y N With x-rays? Y N

Was this appointment for a cleaning? Y N   For a filling? Y N

For a root canal? Y N   For a cap? Y N   For an extraction? Y N

Which tooth (teeth) was treated? _____

Results of check-up and x-rays_____

_____

Treatment plan _____

Dentist_____ Date _____

Dentist Address _____ Ph# _____

Was this appointment a regular check-up? Y N With x-rays? Y N

Was this appointment for a cleaning? Y N   For a filling? Y N

For a root canal? Y N   For a cap? Y N   For an extraction? Y N

Which tooth (teeth) was treated? _____

Results of check-up and x-rays_____

_____

Treatment plan _____

Dentist_____ Date _____

Dentist Address _____ Ph# _____

Was this appointment a regular check-up? Y N With x-rays? Y N

Was this appointment for a cleaning? Y N   For a filling? Y N

For a root canal? Y N   For a cap? Y N   For an extraction? Y N

Which tooth (teeth) was treated? _____

Results of check-up and x-rays_____

_____

Treatment plan _____

Dentist_____ Date _____

Dentist Address _____ Ph#_____

Was this appointment a regular check-up? Y N With x-rays? Y N

Was this appointment for a cleaning? Y N   For a filling? Y N

For a root canal? Y N   For a cap? Y N   For an extraction? Y N

Which tooth (teeth) was treated?_____

Results of check-up and x-rays_____

Treatment plan _____

Dentist_____ Date _____

Dentist Address _____ Ph#_____

Was this appointment a regular check-up? Y N With x-rays? Y N

Was this appointment for a cleaning? Y N   For a filling? Y N

For a root canal? Y N   For a cap? Y N   For an extraction? Y N

Which tooth (teeth) was treated?_____

Results of check-up and x-rays_____

Treatment plan _____

Dentist_____ Date _____

Dentist Address _____ Ph#_____

Was this appointment a regular check-up? Y N With x-rays? Y N

Was this appointment for a cleaning? Y N   For a filling? Y N

For a root canal? Y N   For a cap? Y N   For an extraction? Y N

Which tooth (teeth) was treated?_____

Results of check-up and x-rays_____

Treatment plan _____

DENTAL SURGERIES

Most people have heard the "fact" that George Washington had wooden teeth. In reality, his dentures featured human teeth, as well as fake teeth made from elephant ivory, hippo tusks, and gold.

https://atooth.com

Surgery _____ Date_____

Oral Surgeon_____ Ph.#_____

Where was surgery performed? _____

Reason for surgery_____

Adverse reaction during or after surgery _____

Prescriptions from surgery _____

Length of recovery from surgery _____

Was surgery successful? _____

Notes _____

Surgery ordered during Dentist visit listed on page_____

Surgery _____ Date_____

Oral Surgeon_____ Ph.#_____

Where was surgery performed? _____

Reason for surgery_____

Adverse reaction during or after surgery _____

Prescriptions from surgery _____

Length of recovery from surgery _____

Was surgery successful? _____

Notes _____

Surgery ordered during Dentist visit listed on page_____

Surgery _____ Date_____

Oral Surgeon_____ Ph.#_____

Where was surgery performed? _____

Reason for surgery_____

Adverse reaction during or after surgery _____

Prescriptions from surgery _____

Length of recovery from surgery _____

Was surgery successful? _____

Notes _____

Surgery ordered during Dentist visit listed on page_____

Surgery _____ Date_____

Oral Surgeon_____ Ph.#_____

Where was surgery performed? _____

Reason for surgery_____

Adverse reaction during or after surgery _____

Prescriptions from surgery _____

Length of recovery from surgery _____

Was surgery successful? _____

Notes _____

Surgery ordered during Dentist visit listed on page_____

Surgery _____ Date_____
Oral Surgeon_____ Ph.#_____
Where was surgery performed? _____

Reason for surgery_____

Adverse reaction during or after surgery _____

Prescriptions from surgery _____

Length of recovery from surgery _____
Was surgery successful? _____
Notes _____

Surgery ordered during Dentist visit listed on page_____

Surgery _____ Date_____
Oral Surgeon_____ Ph.#_____
Where was surgery performed? _____

Reason for surgery_____

Adverse reaction during or after surgery _____

Prescriptions from surgery _____

Length of recovery from surgery _____
Was surgery successful? _____
Notes _____

Surgery ordered during Dentist visit listed on page_____

Surgery _____ Date_____

Oral Surgeon_____ Ph.#_____

Where was surgery performed? _____

Reason for surgery_____

Adverse reaction during or after surgery _____

Prescriptions from surgery _____

Length of recovery from surgery _____

Was surgery successful? _____

Notes _____

Surgery ordered during Dentist visit listed on page_____

Surgery _____ Date_____

Oral Surgeon_____ Ph.#_____

Where was surgery performed? _____

Reason for surgery_____

Adverse reaction during or after surgery _____

Prescriptions from surgery _____

Length of recovery from surgery _____

Was surgery successful? _____

Notes _____

Surgery ordered during Dentist visit listed on page_____

Surgery _____ Date_____

Oral Surgeon_____ Ph.#_____

Where was surgery performed? _____

Reason for surgery_____

Adverse reaction during or after surgery _____

Prescriptions from surgery _____

Length of recovery from surgery _____

Was surgery successful? _____

Notes _____

Surgery ordered during Dentist visit listed on page_____

Surgery _____ Date_____

Oral Surgeon_____ Ph.#_____

Where was surgery performed? _____

Reason for surgery_____

Adverse reaction during or after surgery _____

Prescriptions from surgery _____

Length of recovery from surgery _____

Was surgery successful? _____

Notes _____

Surgery ordered during Dentist visit listed on page_____

Surgery _____ Date_____

Oral Surgeon_____ Ph.#_____

Where was surgery performed? _____

Reason for surgery_____

Adverse reaction during or after surgery _____

Prescriptions from surgery _____

Length of recovery from surgery _____

Was surgery successful? _____

Notes _____

Surgery ordered during Dentist visit listed on page_____

Surgery _____ Date_____

Oral Surgeon_____ Ph.#_____

Where was surgery performed? _____

Reason for surgery_____

Adverse reaction during or after surgery _____

Prescriptions from surgery _____

Length of recovery from surgery _____

Was surgery successful? _____

Notes _____

Surgery ordered during Dentist visit listed on page_____

Surgery _____ Date_____

Oral Surgeon_____ Ph.#_____

Where was surgery performed? _____

Reason for surgery_____

Adverse reaction during or after surgery _____

Prescriptions from surgery _____

Length of recovery from surgery _____

Was surgery successful? _____

Notes _____

Surgery ordered during Dentist visit listed on page_____

Surgery _____ Date_____

Oral Surgeon_____ Ph.#_____

Where was surgery performed? _____

Reason for surgery_____

Adverse reaction during or after surgery _____

Prescriptions from surgery _____

Length of recovery from surgery _____

Was surgery successful? _____

Notes _____

Surgery ordered during Dentist visit listed on page_____

Surgery _____ Date_____

Oral Surgeon_____ Ph.#_____

Where was surgery performed? _____

Reason for surgery_____

Adverse reaction during or after surgery _____

Prescriptions from surgery _____

Length of recovery from surgery _____

Was surgery successful? _____

Notes _____

Surgery ordered during Dentist visit listed on page_____

Surgery _____ Date_____

Oral Surgeon_____ Ph.#_____

Where was surgery performed? _____

Reason for surgery_____

Adverse reaction during or after surgery _____

Prescriptions from surgery _____

Length of recovery from surgery _____

Was surgery successful? _____

Notes _____

Surgery ordered during Dentist visit listed on page_____

DENTAL
Prescriptions

Before Novocain was discovered, the most commonly used local anesthetic was cocaine, which was first introduced as a cure for Civil War soldiers' morphine addictions. Over time, it became evident that cocaine was highly addictive and often toxic, prompting researchers to search for an alternative. Before cocaine, dentists used—believe it or not—large quantities of alcohol.

Date _____

Drug Name _____
Prescribed for _____
Dosage _____ Schedule _____ Pharmacy_____
Did medicine cure the problem? Y N   Would I use it again? Y N
List any side effects _____

This medicine was prescribed during the dentist visit on page_____

Date _____

Drug Name _____
Prescribed for _____
Dosage _____ Schedule _____ Pharmacy_____
Did medicine cure the problem? Y N   Would I use it again? Y N
List any side effects _____

This medicine was prescribed during the dentist visit on page_____

Date _____

Drug Name _____
Prescribed for _____
Dosage _____ Schedule _____ Pharmacy_____
Did medicine cure the problem? Y N   Would I use it again? Y N
List any side effects _____

This medicine was prescribed during the dentist visit on page_____

Date _____

Drug Name _____
Prescribed for _____
Dosage _____ Schedule _____ Pharmacy_____
Did medicine cure the problem? Y N   Would I use it again? Y N
List any side effects _____

This medicine was prescribed during the dentist visit on page_____

Date _____

Drug Name _____

Prescribed for _____

Dosage _____ Schedule _____ Pharmacy_____

Did medicine cure the problem? Y N Would I use it again? Y N

List any side effects _____

This medicine was prescribed during the dentist visit on page_____

Date _____

Drug Name _____

Prescribed for _____

Dosage _____ Schedule _____ Pharmacy_____

Did medicine cure the problem? Y N Would I use it again? Y N

List any side effects _____

This medicine was prescribed during the dentist visit on page_____

Date _____

Drug Name _____

Prescribed for _____

Dosage _____ Schedule _____ Pharmacy_____

Did medicine cure the problem? Y N Would I use it again? Y N

List any side effects _____

This medicine was prescribed during the dentist visit on page_____

Date _____

Drug Name _____

Prescribed for _____

Dosage _____ Schedule _____ Pharmacy_____

Did medicine cure the problem? Y N Would I use it again? Y N

List any side effects _____

This medicine was prescribed during the dentist visit on page_____

Date

Drug Name _____

Prescribed for _____

Dosage _____ Schedule _____ Pharmacy_____

Did medicine cure the problem? Y N   Would I use it again? Y   N

List any side effects _____

This medicine was prescribed during the dentist visit on page_____

Date

Drug Name _____

Prescribed for _____

Dosage _____ Schedule _____ Pharmacy_____

Did medicine cure the problem? Y N   Would I use it again? Y   N

List any side effects _____

This medicine was prescribed during the dentist visit on page_____

Date

Drug Name _____

Prescribed for _____

Dosage _____ Schedule _____ Pharmacy_____

Did medicine cure the problem? Y N   Would I use it again? Y   N

List any side effects _____

This medicine was prescribed during the dentist visit on page_____

Date

Drug Name _____

Prescribed for _____

Dosage _____ Schedule _____ Pharmacy_____

Did medicine cure the problem? Y N   Would I use it again? Y   N

List any side effects _____

This medicine was prescribed during the dentist visit on page_____

Date _____

Drug Name _____
Prescribed for _____
Dosage _____ Schedule _____ Pharmacy _____
Did medicine cure the problem? Y N   Would I use it again? Y N
List any side effects _____

This medicine was prescribed during the dentist visit on page _____

Date _____

Drug Name _____
Prescribed for _____
Dosage _____ Schedule _____ Pharmacy _____
Did medicine cure the problem? Y N   Would I use it again? Y N
List any side effects _____

This medicine was prescribed during the dentist visit on page _____

Date _____

Drug Name _____
Prescribed for _____
Dosage _____ Schedule _____ Pharmacy _____
Did medicine cure the problem? Y N   Would I use it again? Y N
List any side effects _____

This medicine was prescribed during the dentist visit on page _____

Date _____

Drug Name _____
Prescribed for _____
Dosage _____ Schedule _____ Pharmacy _____
Did medicine cure the problem? Y N   Would I use it again? Y N
List any side effects _____

This medicine was prescribed during the dentist visit on page _____

Date _____

Drug Name _____

Prescribed for _____

Dosage _____ Schedule _____ Pharmacy _____

Did medicine cure the problem? Y N   Would I use it again? Y N

List any side effects _____

This medicine was prescribed during the dentist visit on page _____

Date _____

Drug Name _____

Prescribed for _____

Dosage _____ Schedule _____ Pharmacy _____

Did medicine cure the problem? Y N   Would I use it again? Y N

List any side effects _____

This medicine was prescribed during the dentist visit on page _____

Date _____

Drug Name _____

Prescribed for _____

Dosage _____ Schedule _____ Pharmacy _____

Did medicine cure the problem? Y N   Would I use it again? Y N

List any side effects _____

This medicine was prescribed during the dentist visit on page _____

Date _____

Drug Name _____

Prescribed for _____

Dosage _____ Schedule _____ Pharmacy _____

Did medicine cure the problem? Y N   Would I use it again? Y N

List any side effects _____

This medicine was prescribed during the dentist visit on page _____

Date _____

Drug Name _____

Prescribed for _____

Dosage _____ Schedule _____ Pharmacy _____

Did medicine cure the problem? Y N   Would I use it again? Y N

List any side effects _____

This medicine was prescribed during the dentist visit on page _____

Date _____

Drug Name _____

Prescribed for _____

Dosage _____ Schedule _____ Pharmacy _____

Did medicine cure the problem? Y N   Would I use it again? Y N

List any side effects _____

This medicine was prescribed during the dentist visit on page _____

Date _____

Drug Name _____

Prescribed for _____

Dosage _____ Schedule _____ Pharmacy _____

Did medicine cure the problem? Y N   Would I use it again? Y N

List any side effects _____

This medicine was prescribed during the dentist visit on page _____

Date _____

Drug Name _____

Prescribed for _____

Dosage _____ Schedule _____ Pharmacy _____

Did medicine cure the problem? Y N   Would I use it again? Y N

List any side effects _____

This medicine was prescribed during the dentist visit on page _____

Date _____

Drug Name _____
Prescribed for _____
Dosage _____ Schedule _____ Pharmacy _____
Did medicine cure the problem? Y N   Would I use it again? Y N
List any side effects _____

This medicine was prescribed during the dentist visit on page _____

Date _____

Drug Name _____
Prescribed for _____
Dosage _____ Schedule _____ Pharmacy _____
Did medicine cure the problem? Y N   Would I use it again? Y N
List any side effects _____

This medicine was prescribed during the dentist visit on page _____

Date _____

Drug Name _____
Prescribed for _____
Dosage _____ Schedule _____ Pharmacy _____
Did medicine cure the problem? Y N   Would I use it again? Y N
List any side effects _____

This medicine was prescribed during the dentist visit on page _____

Date _____

Drug Name _____
Prescribed for _____
Dosage _____ Schedule _____ Pharmacy _____
Did medicine cure the problem? Y N   Would I use it again? Y N
List any side effects _____

This medicine was prescribed during the dentist visit on page _____

Date _____

Drug Name _____
Prescribed for _____
Dosage _____ Schedule _____ Pharmacy _____
Did medicine cure the problem? Y N Would I use it again? Y N
List any side effects _____

This medicine was prescribed during the dentist visit on page _____

Date _____

Drug Name _____
Prescribed for _____
Dosage _____ Schedule _____ Pharmacy _____
Did medicine cure the problem? Y N Would I use it again? Y N
List any side effects _____

This medicine was prescribed during the dentist visit on page _____

Date _____

Drug Name _____
Prescribed for _____
Dosage _____ Schedule _____ Pharmacy _____
Did medicine cure the problem? Y N Would I use it again? Y N
List any side effects _____

This medicine was prescribed during the dentist visit on page _____

Date _____

Drug Name _____
Prescribed for _____
Dosage _____ Schedule _____ Pharmacy _____
Did medicine cure the problem? Y N Would I use it again? Y N
List any side effects _____

This medicine was prescribed during the dentist visit on page _____

Date _____

Drug Name _____
Prescribed for _____
Dosage _____ Schedule _____ Pharmacy_____
Did medicine cure the problem? Y N Would I use it again? Y N
List any side effects _____

This medicine was prescribed during the dentist visit on page_____

Date _____

Drug Name _____
Prescribed for _____
Dosage _____ Schedule _____ Pharmacy_____
Did medicine cure the problem? Y N Would I use it again? Y N
List any side effects _____

This medicine was prescribed during the dentist visit on page_____

Date _____

Drug Name _____
Prescribed for _____
Dosage _____ Schedule _____ Pharmacy_____
Did medicine cure the problem? Y N Would I use it again? Y N
List any side effects _____

This medicine was prescribed during the dentist visit on page_____

Date _____

Drug Name _____
Prescribed for _____
Dosage _____ Schedule _____ Pharmacy_____
Did medicine cure the problem? Y N Would I use it again? Y N
List any side effects _____

This medicine was prescribed during the dentist visit on page_____

Date _____

Drug Name _____

Prescribed for _____

Dosage _____ Schedule _____ Pharmacy _____

Did medicine cure the problem? Y N   Would I use it again? Y N

List any side effects _____

This medicine was prescribed during the dentist visit on page _____

Date _____

Drug Name _____

Prescribed for _____

Dosage _____ Schedule _____ Pharmacy _____

Did medicine cure the problem? Y N   Would I use it again? Y N

List any side effects _____

This medicine was prescribed during the dentist visit on page _____

Date _____

Drug Name _____

Prescribed for _____

Dosage _____ Schedule _____ Pharmacy _____

Did medicine cure the problem? Y N   Would I use it again? Y N

List any side effects _____

This medicine was prescribed during the dentist visit on page _____

Date _____

Drug Name _____

Prescribed for _____

Dosage _____ Schedule _____ Pharmacy _____

Did medicine cure the problem? Y N   Would I use it again? Y N

List any side effects _____

This medicine was prescribed during the dentist visit on page _____

EYE CARE

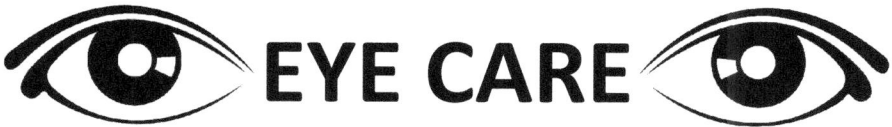

Interesting Facts
about your eyes

1. Your eyes focus on 50 different objects every second.
2. The only organ more complex than the eye is the brain.
3. Your eyes can distinguish approximately 10 million different colors.
4. It is impossible to sneeze with your eyes open.
5. 80 percent of all learning comes through the eyes.
6. Your eyes can detect a candle flame 1.7 miles away.
7. Your iris (the colored part of your eye) has 256 unique characteristics; your fingerprint has just 40.

https://versanthealth.com/blog/15-facts-about-all-things-eyes/

Doctor _____ Date _____

Doctor's Address_____ Ph# _____

Was this appointment a regular check-up?   Y N

Results of appointment _____

Doctor _____ Date _____

Doctor's Address_____ Ph# _____

Was this appointment a regular check-up?   Y N

Results of appointment _____

Doctor _____ Date _____

Doctor's Address_____ Ph# _____

Was this appointment a regular check-up?   Y N

Results of appointment _____

Doctor _____ Date _____

Doctor's Address_____ Ph# _____

Was this appointment a regular check-up?   Y N

Results of appointment _____

Doctor _____ Date _____

Doctor's Address_____ Ph# _____

Was this appointment a regular check-up?   Y N

Results of appointment _____

Doctor _____ Date _____

Doctor's Address_____ Ph# _____

Was this appointment a regular check-up? Y N

Results of appointment _____

_____

Doctor _____ Date _____

Doctor's Address_____ Ph# _____

Was this appointment a regular check-up? Y N

Results of appointment _____

_____

Doctor _____ Date _____

Doctor's Address_____ Ph# _____

Was this appointment a regular check-up? Y N

Results of appointment _____

_____

Doctor _____ Date _____

Doctor's Address_____ Ph# _____

Was this appointment a regular check-up? Y N

Results of appointment _____

_____

Doctor _____ Date _____

Doctor's Address_____ Ph# _____

Was this appointment a regular check-up? Y N

Results of appointment _____

_____

Doctor _____ Date _____

Doctor's Address_____ Ph#_____

Was this appointment a regular check-up?   Y N

Results of appointment _____

Doctor _____ Date _____

Doctor's Address_____ Ph#_____

Was this appointment a regular check-up?   Y N

Results of appointment _____

Doctor _____ Date _____

Doctor's Address_____ Ph#_____

Was this appointment a regular check-up?   Y N

Results of appointment _____

Doctor _____ Date _____

Doctor's Address_____ Ph#_____

Was this appointment a regular check-up?   Y N

Results of appointment _____

Doctor _____ Date _____

Doctor's Address_____ Ph#_____

Was this appointment a regular check-up?   Y N

Results of appointment _____

Doctor _____ Date _____

Doctor's Address_____ Ph# _____

Was this appointment a regular check-up?   Y N

Results of appointment _____

_____

Doctor _____ Date _____

Doctor's Address_____ Ph# _____

Was this appointment a regular check-up?   Y N

Results of appointment _____

_____

Doctor _____ Date _____

Doctor's Address_____ Ph# _____

Was this appointment a regular check-up?   Y N

Results of appointment _____

_____

Doctor _____ Date _____

Doctor's Address_____ Ph# _____

Was this appointment a regular check-up?   Y N

Results of appointment _____

_____

Doctor _____ Date _____

Doctor's Address_____ Ph# _____

Was this appointment a regular check-up?   Y N

Results of appointment _____

_____

Doctor _____ Date _____

Doctor's Address_____ Ph#_____

Was this appointment a regular check-up?   Y   N

Results of appointment _____

_____

Doctor _____ Date _____

Doctor's Address_____ Ph#_____

Was this appointment a regular check-up?   Y   N

Results of appointment _____

_____

Doctor _____ Date _____

Doctor's Address_____ Ph#_____

Was this appointment a regular check-up?   Y   N

Results of appointment _____

_____

Doctor _____ Date _____

Doctor's Address_____ Ph#_____

Was this appointment a regular check-up?   Y   N

Results of appointment _____

_____

Doctor _____ Date _____

Doctor's Address_____ Ph#_____

Was this appointment a regular check-up?   Y   N

Results of appointment _____

_____

Doctor _____ Date _____

Doctor's Address_____ Ph# _____

Was this appointment a regular check-up? Y N

Results of appointment _____

_____

Doctor _____ Date _____

Doctor's Address_____ Ph# _____

Was this appointment a regular check-up? Y N

Results of appointment _____

_____

Doctor _____ Date _____

Doctor's Address_____ Ph# _____

Was this appointment a regular check-up? Y N

Results of appointment _____

_____

Doctor _____ Date _____

Doctor's Address_____ Ph# _____

Was this appointment a regular check-up? Y N

Results of appointment _____

_____

Doctor _____ Date _____

Doctor's Address_____ Ph# _____

Was this appointment a regular check-up? Y N

Results of appointment _____

_____

EYE GLASSES
and Contacts

The earliest known example of wearable eyeglasses dates back to 13th century Italy. A man by the name of Salvino D'Armate is credited with their invention.
https://designeroptics.com/blogs/news/8-fascinating-facts-about-glasses

The first contact lens was designed by Leonardo da Vinci in 1508. But his idea of wearing a water-filled glass hemisphere over the eye was obviously impractical. In 1636, French philosopher Rene Descartes expounded on the idea and proposed a glass tube to be worn directly on the cornea. But because it blocked the eye from blinking, this "contact lens" was also never produced. It took until 1888 for the first fitted contact lens (made from blown glass) to be tolerated, constructed by Adolf Fick, a German ophthalmologist. https://www.professionalvisioncareinc.com/

Optometrist_____ Date _____

Optometrist address_____

Prescription _____

Eye glasses? Y N   Contact lenses? Y N   Both? Y N

Glasses/Contacts purchased at _____

Address_____

Contact Brand_____ Type_____Qty._____

Would you return to this doctor or optical retailer? _____

Optometrist_____ Date _____

Optometrist address_____

Prescription _____

Eye glasses? Y N   Contact lenses? Y N   Both? Y N

Glasses/Contacts purchased at _____

Address_____

Contact Brand_____ Type_____Qty._____

Would you return to this doctor or optical retailer? _____

Optometrist_____ Date _____

Optometrist address_____

Prescription _____

Eye glasses? Y N   Contact lenses? Y N   Both? Y N

Glasses/Contacts purchased at _____

Address_____

Contact Brand_____ Type_____Qty._____

Would you return to this doctor or optical retailer? _____

Optometrist_____ Date _____
Optometrist address_____
Prescription _____
Eye glasses? Y N   Contact lenses? Y N   Both? Y N
Glasses/Contacts purchased at _____
Address_____
Contact Brand_____ Type_____Qty._____
Would you return to this doctor or optical retailer? _____

Optometrist_____ Date _____
Optometrist address_____
Prescription _____
Eye glasses? Y N   Contact lenses? Y N   Both? Y N
Glasses/Contacts purchased at _____
Address_____
Contact Brand_____ Type_____Qty._____
Would you return to this doctor or optical retailer? _____

Optometrist_____ Date _____
Optometrist address_____
Prescription _____
Eye glasses? Y N   Contact lenses? Y N   Both? Y N
Glasses/Contacts purchased at _____
Address_____
Contact Brand_____ Type_____Qty._____
Would you return to this doctor or optical retailer? _____

Optometrist_____ Date _____
Optometrist address_____
Prescription _____
Eye glasses? Y N   Contact lenses? Y N   Both? Y N
Glasses/Contacts purchased at _____
Address_____
Contact Brand_____ Type_____ Qty._____
Would you return to this doctor or optical retailer? _____

Optometrist_____ Date _____
Optometrist address_____
Prescription _____
Eye glasses? Y N   Contact lenses? Y N   Both? Y N
Glasses/Contacts purchased at _____
Address_____
Contact Brand_____ Type_____ Qty._____
Would you return to this doctor or optical retailer? _____

Optometrist_____ Date _____
Optometrist address_____
Prescription _____
Eye glasses? Y N   Contact lenses? Y N   Both? Y N
Glasses/Contacts purchased at _____
Address_____
Contact Brand_____ Type_____ Qty._____
Would you return to this doctor or optical retailer? _____

Optometrist_____ Date _____

Optometrist address_____

Prescription _____

Eye glasses? Y N   Contact lenses? Y N   Both? Y N

Glasses/Contacts purchased at _____

Address_____

Contact Brand_____ Type_____ Qty._____

Would you return to this doctor or optical retailer? _____

Optometrist_____ Date _____

Optometrist address_____

Prescription _____

Eye glasses? Y N   Contact lenses? Y N   Both? Y N

Glasses/Contacts purchased at _____

Address_____

Contact Brand_____ Type_____ Qty._____

Would you return to this doctor or optical retailer? _____

Optometrist_____ Date _____

Optometrist address_____

Prescription _____

Eye glasses? Y N   Contact lenses? Y N   Both? Y N

Glasses/Contacts purchased at _____

Address_____

Contact Brand_____ Type_____ Qty._____

Would you return to this doctor or optical retailer? _____

Optometrist_____ Date _____

Optometrist address_____

Prescription _____

Eye glasses? Y N   Contact lenses? Y N   Both? Y N

Glasses/Contacts purchased at _____

Address_____

Contact Brand_____ Type_____Qty._____

Would you return to this doctor or optical retailer? _____

Optometrist_____ Date _____

Optometrist address_____

Prescription _____

Eye glasses? Y N   Contact lenses? Y N   Both? Y N

Glasses/Contacts purchased at _____

Address_____

Contact Brand_____ Type_____Qty._____

Would you return to this doctor or optical retailer? _____

Optometrist_____ Date _____

Optometrist address_____

Prescription _____

Eye glasses? Y N   Contact lenses? Y N   Both? Y N

Glasses/Contacts purchased at _____

Address_____

Contact Brand_____ Type_____Qty._____

Would you return to this doctor or optical retailer? _____

Optometrist_____ Date _____

Optometrist address_____

Prescription _____

Eye glasses? Y N   Contact lenses? Y N   Both? Y N

Glasses/Contacts purchased at _____

Address_____

Contact Brand_____ Type_____ Qty._____

Would you return to this doctor or optical retailer? _____

Optometrist_____ Date _____

Optometrist address_____

Prescription _____

Eye glasses? Y N   Contact lenses? Y N   Both? Y N

Glasses/Contacts purchased at _____

Address_____

Contact Brand_____ Type_____ Qty._____

Would you return to this doctor or optical retailer? _____

Optometrist_____ Date _____

Optometrist address_____

Prescription _____

Eye glasses? Y N   Contact lenses? Y N   Both? Y N

Glasses/Contacts purchased at _____

Address_____

Contact Brand_____ Type_____ Qty._____

Would you return to this doctor or optical retailer? _____

EYE SURGERIES

The origins of cataract surgery are embedded in antiquity, with the very first procedures performed in the fifth century BC. The procedure at the time used a technique called couching, and was performed only in extremely advanced cataracts.

The first true case of cataract surgery was performed by French surgeon Jacques Daviel in Paris in 1747. His procedure was more effective than couching with an overall success rate of 50%. Surgery involved making a large incision around the cornea, through which the intact lens was extracted, leaving at least part of the lens capsule behind. This was a great improvement on couching, but was plagued with postoperative complications, including infection inside the eye.

https://www.nexushospitals.com.au/the-history-of-cataract-surgery/

Surgery _____ Date_____

Surgeon _____ Ph.# _____

Where was surgery performed? _____

Reason for surgery_____

_____

_____

Adverse reaction during or after surgery _____

_____

_____

Length of recovery from surgery _____

Was surgery successful? _____

Surgery ordered during Doctor visit listed on page _____

Surgery _____ Date_____

Surgeon _____ Ph.# _____

Where was surgery performed? _____

Reason for surgery_____

_____

_____

Adverse reaction during or after surgery _____

_____

_____

Length of recovery from surgery _____

Was surgery successful? _____

Surgery ordered during Doctor visit listed on page _____

Surgery _____ Date_____

Surgeon _____ Ph.#_____

Where was surgery performed? _____

Reason for surgery_____

Adverse reaction during or after surgery _____

Length of recovery from surgery _____

Was surgery successful? _____

Surgery ordered during Doctor visit listed on page _____

Surgery _____ Date_____

Surgeon _____ Ph.#_____

Where was surgery performed? _____

Reason for surgery_____

Adverse reaction during or after surgery _____

Length of recovery from surgery _____

Was surgery successful? _____

Surgery ordered during Doctor visit listed on page _____

Surgery _____ Date_____

Surgeon _____ Ph.# _____

Where was surgery performed? _____

Reason for surgery_____

Adverse reaction during or after surgery _____

Length of recovery from surgery _____

Was surgery successful? _____

Surgery ordered during Doctor visit listed on page ____

Surgery _____ Date_____

Surgeon _____ Ph.# _____

Where was surgery performed? _____

Reason for surgery_____

Adverse reaction during or after surgery _____

Length of recovery from surgery _____

Was surgery successful? _____

Surgery ordered during Doctor visit listed on page ____

Surgery _____ Date_____

Surgeon _____ Ph.# _____

Where was surgery performed? _____

Reason for surgery_____

_____

Adverse reaction during or after surgery _____

_____

Length of recovery from surgery _____

Was surgery successful? _____

Surgery ordered during Doctor visit listed on page _____

Surgery _____ Date_____

Surgeon _____ Ph.# _____

Where was surgery performed? _____

Reason for surgery_____

_____

Adverse reaction during or after surgery _____

_____

Length of recovery from surgery _____

Was surgery successful? _____

Surgery ordered during Doctor visit listed on page _____

Surgery _____ Date_____

Surgeon _____ Ph.# _____

Where was surgery performed? _____

Reason for surgery_____

_____

Adverse reaction during or after surgery _____

_____

Length of recovery from surgery _____

Was surgery successful? _____

Surgery ordered during Doctor visit listed on page _____

Surgery _____ Date_____

Surgeon _____ Ph.# _____

Where was surgery performed? _____

Reason for surgery_____

_____

Adverse reaction during or after surgery _____

_____

Length of recovery from surgery _____

Was surgery successful? _____

Surgery ordered during Doctor visit listed on page _____

Surgery _____ Date_____

Surgeon _____ Ph.# _____

Where was surgery performed? _____

Reason for surgery_____

_____

Adverse reaction during or after surgery _____

_____

Length of recovery from surgery _____

Was surgery successful? _____

Surgery ordered during Doctor visit listed on page _____

Surgery _____ Date_____

Surgeon _____ Ph.# _____

Where was surgery performed? _____

Reason for surgery_____

_____

Adverse reaction during or after surgery _____

_____

Length of recovery from surgery _____

Was surgery successful? _____

Surgery ordered during Doctor visit listed on page _____

NOTES

Use the following pages to make any notes that you find necessary. Remember to reference the page of the doctors visit that the note refers to.

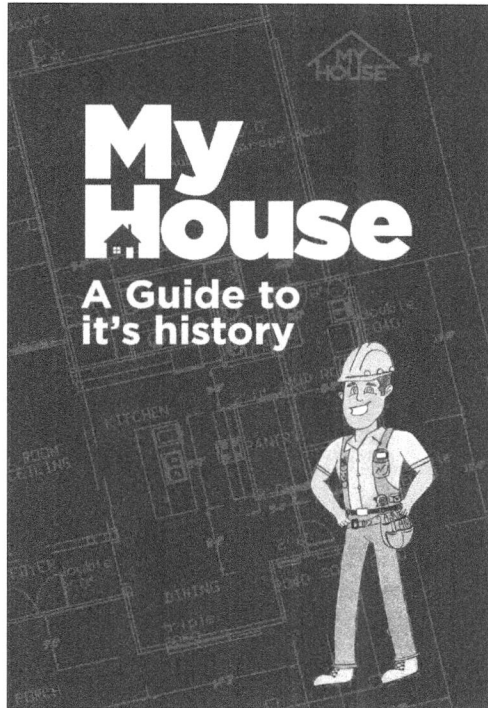

AVAILABLE
From Amazon
$14.99

ISBN
978-1-947729-08-7

MY HOUSE

A comprehensive guide to your home's history, *My House* is a wealth of information at your fingertips. You will always have an accurate record of purchases, repairs, colors, styles and brands of the essential components of your home.

Do you wish you could remember the color you painted the Dining Room five years ago? Or maybe what the brand and color of the carpet in the Master Bedroom is? There is no more guessing with *My House.* All your pertinent information is available at anytime.

And as this book passes from homeowner to homeowner, your home's history will be preserved providing the next owner with valuable and much needed information.

So let's get started writing your home's story for people to read for years to come!